GOAL:
Carryover

GOAL:
Carryover

An Articulation Manual and Program

ADELE GERBER

Temple University Press
Philadelphia

Temple University Press, Philadelphia 19122
©1973 by Temple University
All rights reserved. Published 1973
PRINTED IN THE UNITED STATES OF AMERICA

International Standard Book Number: 0-87722-021-2
Library of Congress Catalog Card Number: 72-95886

CONTENTS

FOREWORD

CARRYOVER may be defined as the realization of a response in novel situations in which it is appropriate but for which there has been no direct training. The achievement of carryover is necessary before any teaching can be considered successful.

The teaching of the appropriate use of the sounds of English (articulation therapy) is no exception; the successful case will show consistent ability to use the correct sound in the appropriate linguistic context and in all speaking situations. But it is apparent that no therapy program could hope to directly teach the correct sounds in all the contexts in which they might appear or in all the speaking situations in which the individual might engage, since the number of these is indeterminately great in their variety.

It is obvious that the individual must learn more than a particular response for a limited range of contexts. He must learn something beyond this that insures the generalization of the response to all contexts in which it is appropriate where appropriateness is determined by a significant similarity between the contexts trained and those that have not been, no matter how different they are in other regards. What must he learn in order to insure carryover? Apparently, he must learn the relevant rule for recognizing the appropriate context whenever it occurs in any of its manifestations. This means that he knows *what* is to be done, what response is called for. Second, he must know how to execute the response when the response itself must vary with context without loss of essential identity. There are, then, two sorts of knowledge or skill the individual must acquire: the ability to recognize the conditions calling for the response, and the ability to appropriately embed that response in its various contexts.

Most of this is roughly understood by all clinicians; nevertheless, they routinely complain about the difficulty of achieving carryover. Specifically, clinicians find it relatively easy to teach production of a sound of English and to teach the use of that sound in a limited range of contexts consisting of the words and sentences worked with in the treatment session. They find, however, that, upon introduction of other linguistic contexts or in the performance of the individual in other speaking situations, the sound is inconsistently employed, if at all. Assuming cooperation and motivation on the part of the client, we must conclude that the clinicians do not know how to teach the client what he needs to know in order to respond appropriately in novel situations.

The present manual provides a principled procedure for insuring carryover in that it gives the client production practice in a variety of phonological contexts and requires him to attend to his performance in contexts and situations in which the response is appropriate. This is exactly what is required to induce those general attributes necessary to the recognition of appropriate context and to acquire those performance skills for embedding the response (sound) in its various contexts. The client, then, is instructed by working on exemplars of phonetic context and by being required to assess his own performance in them. No general rule is ever stated, but the contexts necessary for its appreciation are provided, and he is directed in the proper handling of them.

The techniques in this manual have been used with success by the author, her students, and her immediate colleagues. She has done clinicians and clients elsewhere a service by making them available through this publication.

HENRY GOEHL

Professor of Speech
Temple University

PREFACE

THIS manual is concerned with the achievement of carryover of corrected articulation to spontaneous speech. With one exception, it does not address itself to the acquisition stage of articulation modification, since I believe that the literature in speech pathology provides a relatively large body of information, both theoretical and practical, devoted to the acquisition of target sounds. To the present time, however, little has been published in the area of carryover. Yet this aspect of therapy continues to present vexing problems to both clinician and client, contributing in a large measure to the protracted nature of the correction process.

In a survey of 176 speech clinicians in Pennsylvania, working in public schools, hospitals, and university clinics, more than 75 percent of the respondents ranked carryover as the problem presenting the greatest difficulty in articulation therapy (Sommers 1969, pp. 307–9).

The stages of articulation therapy have been characterized as acquisition, generalization, and automatization (Wright, Shelton, and Arndt 1969). The program described herein is designed for that phase of training which follows acquisition of the target sound, proceeding from that point of essential but minimal skill through a step-by-step progression toward the ultimate goal of automatization. The criterion in the program, which I have arbitrarily established, is from 90 to 100 percent correct production of the target sound in a communicative situation wherein the client's attention is focused on the content of the message and not on the deliberate control of the mechanics of speech production.

The present manual is divided into three parts: Part I contains an account of the development of the rationale for the approach to articulation therapy presented herein; Part II presents material and procedures appropriate for use with any sound; Part III is devoted exclusively to a program of [r] therapy. The latter program has been developed as a separate entity because correction of defective [r] seems to present unique problems that require unique treatment.

It should be noted that the methods herein presented are not necessarily advocated for use in all cases of all ages. Clinical experience has confirmed the validity of the recommendations in the literature for a less direct approach for young children within the speech development stage. For the child under approximately seven years of age, the developmental processes are apparently amenable to stimulation through heightened auditory perception in conjunction with sound production in communicative units. During this period and by means of such procedures, the relatively plastic organism appears capable of incorporating modifications of speech patterns at a level below that of volitional, structured correction. When training can be conducted without fractionation, results may frequently be achieved less laboriously and more rapidly.

For the older child, in whom maturational processes are no longer functioning to the same degree and whose defective speech patterns are more rigidly established, a more direct and fractionated approach has usually been found necessary. The program presented herein represents the latter approach. It has been used with hundreds of school-age children (and, in modified form, with adults) and has been found effective.

The structured nature of the program reflects my analysis of the processes and levels of processes involved in the progress toward achievement of the terminal objective. All clients may not require all activities at all levels. For those who do, the full range of materials, systematically ordered, is available. The degree to which they are used and the nature of the selection for each client depend upon the discretion of the clinician.

I hope that the use of these materials, based upon an understanding of their rationale, will be helpful to clinicians in the achievement of carryover of corrected articulation to spontaneous speech.

ADELE GERBER

I

INTRODUCTION

1

EVOLUTION OF THE RATIONALE

THIS manual consists of a program of clinically tested materials and procedures and the rationale upon which that program is constructed. The program is different in certain major aspects from many widely used methods of articulation modification, the difference having developed as the result of a combination of factors: intensive clinical experience with articulation problems, effective supervision, and certain key contributions from the literature. A thorough understanding of the rationale, prerequisite to effective use of the materials, can probably be best developed by means of an account of how the present program evolved.

The impetus for change grew as the result of frustration experienced in attempts to get clients to achieve carryover of corrected speech sounds into truly spontaneous speech by means of certain commonly employed practices. Initially, the Van Riper method was faithfully adhered to. Ear training was followed by sound production and stabilization in isolation. The nonsense syllable was employed until the sound was consistently correct under conditions of careful control in the initial, medial, and final positions. Next, the sound was elicited in words, phrases,

3

and sentences on the assumption that the sooner corrected production was incorporated into meaningful context, the sooner carryover would occur.

However, in case after case, it became evident that the newly acquired sound was produced in connected speech only under conditions of careful control. When attention shifted to the content of the message in truly spontaneous speech, the old error patterns inevitably appeared and remained strongly resistant to change. This baffling phenomenon gave rise to the question, "How can I get the client to slow down his spontaneous speech to the point at which he can give careful attention to the production of his newly acquired sound?" Such an approach to the problem was of course doomed to failure, since spontaneous speech slowed to the careful level is no longer spontaneous. After continued frustration, it eventually became apparent that a solution was possible only if the question was changed to, "How can I get the client to produce the corrected sound in the rapid, automatic manner characteristic of spontaneous speech?"

The first departure from the previously described approach was made at the suggestion of Ronald K. Sommers, then supervisor of the public school program within which I was functioning. He suggested that the use of meaningful words be deferred to permit greater exploitation of the nonsense syllable. Implementation of this recommendation resulted in the design of a variety of procedures aimed at the client's ability to produce the target sound in simple CV, VCV, and VC syllables at increasingly rapid rates of speed while maintaining a high degree of consistency.

The realization of this goal made a contribution to the achievement of effortless articulation as a result of the reduction of laborious exaggeration in production of the corrected sound. Some gain in carryover was noted. However, it was observed that a high degree of error persisted on sounds in unstressed words, particularly in small functor words of relatively little communicative content.

Strategies to cope with this problem were stimulated by the McDonald (1964) approach, which utilized shifting stress patterns in practice sentences. The concept was adapted to the development of structured drills incorporating the target sound in many combinations of stressed-unstressed syllables, to be produced, as a result of practice, at the speed of ongoing speech. Such procedures, in addition to the speed drills on equally stressed syllables mentioned above, further deferred the introduction of meaningful material.

Another major contribution was made by Shames (1957) on the use of the nonsense syllable in articulation therapy. As a result of his concern with the gap between deliberate and automatic sound production, he investigated factors interfering with the transfer of newly acquired sounds to spontaneous communication. Clients questioned about the interference reported that, although they had been admonished to "slow down enough to put the new sound in," the need to control rate and to concentrate on sound production distracted them from the content of their ideas and distorted phrasing and inflection patterns to the point of rendering communication artificial and lacking in satisfaction.

Shames concluded that there was a need to develop newly acquired skills to the point of automaticity before aiming at their use communicatively. He considered the function of the jargon phase of speech development as the period during which the child's newly acquired repertoire of phonemes is practiced in various rates, rhythms, and inflection patterns. This led to the concept of including such a stage in the learning of new articulatory patterns during the therapy process. He devised a structured jargon technique which provided intensive practice of the new sound by substituting nonsense syllables for actual words in a passage. The rate, phrasing, and intonation patterns appropriate to the meaningful material were incorporated into the syllable jargon. This bridging of the gap between deliberate and automatic speech was reported to result in "an immediate and automatic carryover into reading and talking."

Shames' rationale and procedures gave further impetus to the development of a diverse repertoire of nonsense materials, the manipulation of which gave rise to the evolution of an increasingly refined set of subgoals. The principle of overlapping articulatory gestures involved in the production of abutting consonants, exemplified in McDonald's Deep Test and Treatment program, was applied to the construction of lists of nonsense words of specifically tailored phonetic complexity. These were designed to take into consideration both the articulatory dynamics of the target sound and the needs of the individual client. Skill in the production of the newly acquired sound in controlled complex phonetic environments made another contribution to the ability to utter the corrected sound within the stream of running speech.

The principles emerging from this background are further explored and discussed in the next chapter in the light of their application to the procedures of the present program.

2

PRINCIPLES AND PROCEDURES

C AREFUL, deliberate utterance of modified sounds appears to be necessary at certain stages of acquisition if correct production is to be achieved. This type of behavior is reported in the literature and observed clinically. It cannot be conclusively determined here whether this phenomenon is the result of "interference from the old articulatory response" (Winitz 1969), as a result of "competition of the old error" (Van Riper 1963), or whether it occurs as a function of focusing attention on an individual sound within a word instead of on the word as a meaningful whole. The behavior, which may be accounted for by any, all, or none of the above explanations, seems to be indispensable to the disruption of established patterns and the production and conscious monitoring of new speech sounds. However, the undue persistence of this mode of corrected production appears to interfere with the achievement of carryover to spontaneous speech, since the latter is characterized by neither careful attention to, nor deliberate production of, the individual sounds which transmit the spoken message. It is quite evident that deliberate speech and automatic speech constitute two distinctly different levels (and—perhaps—kinds) of behavior.

Therefore, the overriding principle determining the procedures

6

of this program is that bridging the gap between these disparate modes of speech behavior is imperative. The attributes of the terminal behavior—that is, spontaneous, running speech—should be the constant objectives of the processes in which clinician and client are mutually engaged. These attributes should be clearly perceived in the formulation and attainment of each of the subgoals in the sequence leading cumulatively to the desired competence. Elicitation and reinforcement of responses which do not promote progress toward the achievement of those attributes would appear to be counterproductive. Therefore, if training is to be efficient and effective, it is important for the clinician to analyze the characteristics of the terminal behavior and, in the light of this analysis, to evaluate the efficacy of responses to certain classes of stimuli employed in the clinical situation.

CONTRASTIVE ANALYSIS OF THE ATTRIBUTES OF SPONTANEOUS AND STRUCTURED SPEECH

Spontaneous Speech	Structured Speech
Articulatory movements are rapidly overlapping and effortless	Articulatory movements are frequently artificially prolonged and strenuous.
Articulation is subordinated in consciousness to the content of the message; therefore, production is relatively automatic	Attention is focused on the mechanics of sound production; therefore, production is deliberate, frequently emitted from a preparatory set.
Segmental sounds are modified by natural patterns of stress, juncture, and intonation related to meaning.	Stress patterns are frequently distorted through exaggerated production. Rhythm and melody are often stilted and artificial.

Since it appears that premature attempts to produce altered sound patterns in familiar words frequently result in conscious, belabored articulation, and since it is believed that early achievement of consistently effortless production of the new patterns facilitates carryover, meaningful speech is withheld until production of the target sound is possible under conditions of running speech.

This principle and its accompanying practice receive support from Van Riper (1963) and Winitz (1969). Van Riper reasons that the advantage of using nonsense material is that no unlearning is required. He recommends a variety of ways in which this material can be manipulated in pseudocommunicative contexts, in a variety of phonetic combinations, and at increasing rates of speed.

Winitz advocates what he calls an intensive period of pretraining with nonsense material, stating: "Finally, when the sounds within the nonsense words are highly learned in connected speech, a few English words are introduced. Generalization of the newly learned sounds in English words should then occur more rapidly than if the nonsense pre-training had not been done."

The Winitz text contains an exhaustive treatment of the theory and research findings related to this topic.

In the present program, nonsense materials conforming to the permissible phonological patterns of English are arranged in the following hierarchy of complexity:

1. Simple CV, VCV, and VC syllables.
2. More complex syllables, including, where appropriate, consonant clusters in the releasing, arresting, and intervocalic position.
   CCV   VCCV   VCC.
3. Simple nonsense words.
   CVC.
4. More complex nonsense words specifically tailored to meet the client's needs.
   Multisyllabic configurations: e.g., sikesoo, lanasos.
   Variations in abutting consonants in releasing and
   arresting positions: e.g., kapset, kikso.
5. "Phrases" composed of nonsense words.
   Examples are presented in the program material.
6. "Conversations" in nonsense words.
   Examples are presented in the program material.
7. Embedding nonsense material in meaningful units.
   Examples are presented in the program material.

The visual representation of the syllables in practice material for young children has presented problems due to the lack of a one-to-one correspondence between phoneme and grapheme in written English. Since the primary purpose of these syllables is to elicit rapid, effortless speech, it was found necessary to circumvent the intricacies of vowel phonics to the greatest extent possible. Rather than resort to the various digraphs employed orthographically to represent the long vowels occurring in open CV syllables, thereby requiring the beginning reader to engage in a relatively complex process of decoding, I have used a device calling for the consistent application of only one rule: when you see a letter say its name. Only a minor adjustment for the "u" is required. For complete consistency, this system has been extended to other environments (VC; VCV). Although, admittedly, this system violates phonic rules, virtually all children using the materials have been able to separate the system employed for speech drills from the rules related to bona fide reading.

Choice of the releasing, arresting, or intervocalic position of the target consonant, for the purpose of preliminary stabilization, is made at the discretion of the clinician, depending on the nature of the sound and the problems the client has in effecting transition to or from the vowel. For example, it has been found that lateral lispers can more easily maintain central emission when moving to the sibilant from the vowel, whereas interdental lispers appear to have greater success by moving from the new consonant position to the vowel.

In accordance with the previously stated principle, each level of nonsense material is programmed, in a gradual progression, to achieve production characterized by the attributes of running speech. Beginning at a point which insures greatest probability of success, these subgoals are arranged in levels that are minimally incremental in difficulty and cumulative in effect. Thus, the above levels of nonsense material are practiced to attain the following attributes:

1. Consistency of target sound production.
   (This is usually performed at a slow, careful rate, sometimes, when necessary, separating consonant and vowel.)
2. Consistency plus connection.
   (Production is characterized by smooth transition between consonant and vowel and, ultimately, multiple utterances on one breath.)
3. Consistency plus connection plus speed.
   (Hitting the target on the run achieves effortless, unexaggerated production.)
4. Consistency plus connection plus speed plus unstress.
   (Correct production is maintained on syllables of reduced duration and loudness and lowered pitch.)
5. Consistency plus connection plus speed plus unstress plus phonetic complexity.
   (Correct production is maintained in systematically varied phonetic environments, in wordlike configurations.)
6. Consistency plus connection plus speed plus unstress plus phonetic complexity plus syntactic structure.
   (Correct production is maintained in pseudosentences— i.e., utterances characterized by natural intonational contours and reduced meaningful content.)

Only after the target sound has been produced under all of the above conditions is the introduction of meaningful material recommended. At this point, correct production without undue effort is virtually guaranteed, thereby increasing the likelihood that the sound can be uttered in a word or sentence without preparatory set and exaggerated articulation. Thus, embedding the corrected sound in passages of meaningful running speech can be accomplished at a level of automaticity which permits maximal focusing of attention on the content with a minimum of distraction by the mechanics of articulation.

This level of mastery cannot be achieved unless the client "has passed through a period during which he was willing and able to pay conscious attention to the sound of his own speech" (Carrell 1968). In order to achieve the goal of carryover, it has been found that self-monitoring skills require systematic training that is as carefully programmed as the training of articulatory gestures. As the goals for production are set at successively higher levels of speed and complexity, the ability to attend to auditory, visual, and proprioceptive cues must be trained to keep apace, in order to insure self-evaluation under these increasingly demanding conditions.

The practice of rewarding accurate self-evaluation of both correct and incorrect productions can provide two important benefits. On each trial, the client may experience a success even though he may have failed to achieve target production, and, cumulatively, he achieves a highly refined degree of precision in self-monitoring. This precision can be achieved by starting with easy behavior (i.e., evaluating specific aspects of a model's production) and moving in a step-by-step progression to the difficult behavior (i.e., evaluating aspects of one's own speech behavior).

A detailed program of training in self-evaluation is presented below in Chapter 7. Whereas the procedures outlined there focus primary attention on auditory cues, the same or similar techniques can be employed to intensify visual, tactile, and kinesthetic feedback. The two key factors around which the auditory self-monitoring program was constructed are precision and hierarchical levels of difficulty. The procedures and the levels in the auditory training procedures can be adapted to whatever additional modalities may require training to achieve appropriate monitoring of specific target productions.

II

AN APPROACH TO
CONSONANT SOUND CORRECTION

3

THE PROGRAM

THE materials in this program were designed to provide a high target-response rate, to foster a high level of motivation, to stimulate specific goal-seeking behavior, and to create an awareness of visible progress.

It is generally acknowledged that extensive practice of the target sounds is required to eliminate habitual error patterns and to establish new articulation skills. It is also recognized that unrelieved, unmotivated, and unrewarding drill will usually result in boredom and diminished effort. Attempting to resolve this dilemma, speech clinicians have frequently resorted to the device of game therapy in order to generate enthusiastic participation. However, this approach has come under sharp attack recently from a number of sources on the grounds that it does not provide the most efficient means of speech behavior modification.

John Irwin, in a 1967 address in Montgomery County, Pennsylvania, stated that articulation therapy should be kept at a level just above that of boredom. Since the details of behavior the client must be trained to observe, modify, monitor, and control are not generally readily perceptible, in addition to usually being highly resistant to change, keen attention and refined evaluation are required to effect correction. Game therapy, by virtue of its diverting nature, tends to distract attention from the crucial details of speech behavior to aspects of the game activity.

In addition, the uneconomical use of therapy time spent in games drastically reduces the opportunity for practice of the target patterns. Mowrer et al. (1968), as the result of analyses of the utilization of time during speech therapy sessions, found, among other things, that "an average child in group therapy produced the target sound only one half of one percent of the speaking time." Results of further investigations by Mowrer (1970) suggest that increased response rate and increased response accuracy are related to successful instructional techniques. He strongly recommends that those aspects of therapy which tend to reduce response rate should be eliminated from the procedures.

The materials in the present program do afford the client the opportunity for many productions of the target sound. The technique employed might be described as halfway between that used in game therapy and that used in operant conditioning therapy. In the former approach, enhanced stimuli are predominately instrumental in eliciting the desired behavior. The practice material is disguised in a fashion somewhat analogous to the medicine in a candy-coated pill. In the latter method, stimulus presentation is usually relatively straightforward; reinforcement, contingent on the client's response, is the instrument primarily responsible for increasing emission of the desired behavior. In other words, the "medicine" is administered "straight," and the "candy" follows.

The materials in this manual incorporate the stimulus material, undisguised, in activities designed to arouse interest and require active participation, with the client's attention focused on the quality of the speech production in the performance of a challenging task. Each activity is recognizably different from the others. In contrast to endless, formless drill, each activity has a structure that has a beginning and an end. Each contains enough of a challenge to stimulate repeated effort. The completion of each activity, with the accomplishment of its particular subgoal, moves the client noticeably closer to the achievement of the attributes of the terminal behavior.

While tangible reinforcers may, and frequently should, be used in conjunction with the activities, the self-esteem resulting from gratification of the drive toward mastery has been observed to be a most potent motivating force. Thus, the program attempts to provide both attractive stimuli and built-in rewards for target response emission.

APPLICATION TO GROUP THERAPY

A large part of my early experience was gained in the public school setting, where group therapy is often the method employed. Group articulation therapy can be highly efficacious if maximum advantage is taken of the group interaction without neglecting individual needs. It is most effective when there is a group drive toward goals clearly set by the clinician and clearly perceived by the clients. At times, when appropriate to the level of achievement attained and to the nature of the material, the entire group may work together as a unit. However, some individual work is often indicated, especially in cases where progress of some members has not matched that of others in the group. At these times, other members must be profitably engaged in activities that do more than just keep them busy. The materials in Parts II and III have been designed to serve either as total group activities or as material equally suitable for practice in subgroups while the clinician is engaged with individuals.

One of the criticisms of group work has been that too much of the members' time is spent in waiting for turns, thereby sharply depressing the target response rates and rendering group therapy relatively inefficient. This need not be true if members of the group are trained to serve as "speech aides" for each other, supervising the practice of their peers on assigned materials. If all members have been intensively involved in a group interaction, evaluating each other and providing models for each other, they become keenly attuned to the target behaviors and function as reliable monitors. The structured format of the activities in the present program fosters repeated practice. Competition among members adds additional motivation for self-imposed effort. The hierarchy of activity provides a convenient structure within which the clinician can plan for the clients' progress.

4

THERAPY TECHNIQUES

THE procedures and materials described and illustrated below have been found successful in articulation therapy with clients from primary grades through high school. All are not equally appropriate to all age levels, but, used with discretion, they are adaptable to different age groups. The format is designed to permit use with any sound or sound combinations. The materials are presented with sample drills inserted. The [s] sound is used as illustrative material in the samples. In actual use, the clinician would write practice material suitable to each client's needs in blank forms reproduced by xerography from the master sheets provided with this manual.

The various types of practice material are presented as examples of the ways in which syllables, nonsense words, and so on may be constructed. They are intended to be suggestive rather than prescriptive, since the nature of each articulation problem must determine the composition of the material used in its management.

HOPSCOTCH

Hopscotch, like the frequently used ladder, is a device for motivating consistency in the syllable drill. The index and sec-

16

ond fingers are used as "feet," and either "hop" in the single blocks or "jump" together in the pairs of blocks. The goal is to hop in all the blocks without "stepping on a line" or making an error in production. Should an error be made, the sound is corrected in that block, but the client must start again at the beginning. The purpose is to achieve careful production in an increasingly connected flow of utterance.

Stimulus Materials

1. Use broken syllables in three positions (C-V, V-C-V, V-C), represented by consonant and vowels separated by a hyphen if production has not as yet been achieved in transition to and from the vowel. In fig. 1 only C-V syllables are used. In actual practice the clinician may use other blank sheets for VC and/or VCV syllables.

2. Use connected syllables in three positions (CV, VCV, VC) when production has been correctly achieved in transition to and from the vowel. In fig. 2 only VCV syllables are used. In actual practice the clinician may use other blank sheets for CV and/or VC syllables.

Procedures

1. The clinician writes syllables in the blocks, saying each syllable as it is written. The client imitates the model.

2. The client "hops" with fingers in each block, reading the syllables if possible, imitating the clinician's model if reading is not possible.

3. As a result of frequent repetition, with the assistance of the clinician or another client who can read, the nonreading client eventually memorizes the syllables.

4. After preliminary practice, the client competes with his own past performances, or in a group with other clients, to see how many times he can complete the hopscotch pattern without error, going up and down. A check is placed in the score blocks each time he successfully completes the task. When all of the score blocks are checked, the client proceeds to the next activity.

SOUND HURDLES

The goal in this activity is consistently correct production in syllables with speed. A stopwatch or a watch with a second hand is used to time "contestants" in the race. Production should be continuous and connected, imitating the patterns of running

Score

SOUND HOPSCOTCH

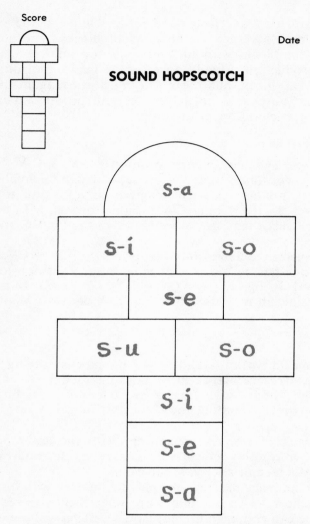

Fig. 1. Sound hopscotch: broken syllables in one position (C-V)

Score

SOUND HOPSCOTCH

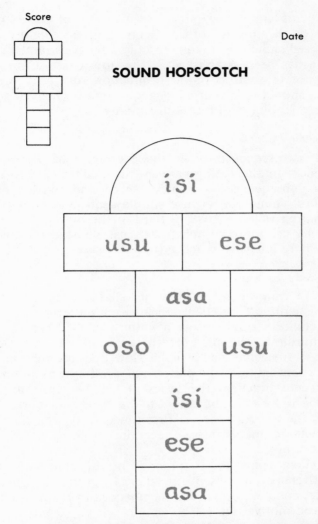

Fig. 2. Sound hopscotch: connected syllables in one position (VCV)

speech. Clients aim to beat their own record of preceding sessions and/or the time of other clients if group therapy is employed. Speed should be attempted only after consistently correct production has been established at the slower rate. Care should be taken not to sacrifice good production for speed. Careless production should be penalized by requiring the client to go back to the starting point with time still running.

Stimulus Materials

Use only two sequences of syllable combinations. Repeat these two sequences in alternating patterns, to facilitate memorization and, as a consequence, to achieve speed and fluency of production. For young clients, use simple sequences composed of two alternating syllables, with a third at the hurdle (fig. 3). For older clients, use more complex patterns. The greater challenge motivates more intensive practice (fig. 4).

Procedures

1. The clinician writes patterns of syllables, saying each syllable as it is written. The client repeats each pattern.

2. The clinician produces each pattern of syllables (sequence between hurdles) on one breath without pausing between syllables. At first, the rate will be slow and production deliberate. The client imitates the patterns as produced by the model.

3. The client practices the series of syllable patterns. When each sequence between hurdles can be produced correctly on one breath, he is ready for his first timed trial. The number of seconds required to complete the entire exercise is marked in the first score box.

4. The client continues to practice in order to improve his own speed record on subsequent trials. In group therapy, when appropriate, competition among members can provide additional challenge and motivation.

RHYTHM DRILLS

Follow the Beat

This activity is used to develop correct production in stressed and unstressed syllables, since spontaneous speech is characterized by such a pattern. Clients are taught to "hit the target" on the little, quick sounds as well as on the long, slow sounds in speech. Children enjoy practicing their syllables in various musical rhythms. Because they find the activity pleasant, it is easy to

SOUND HURDLES

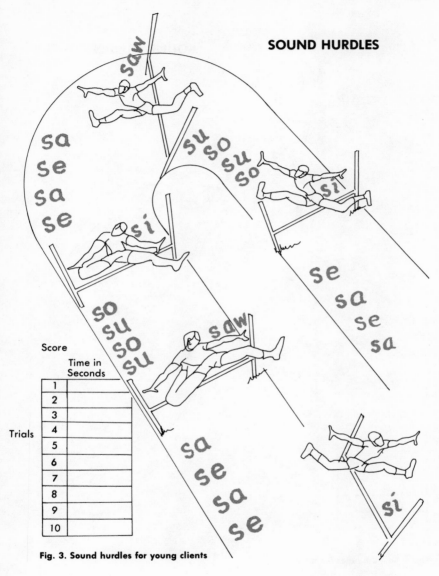

Fig. 3. Sound hurdles for young clients

SOUND HURDLES

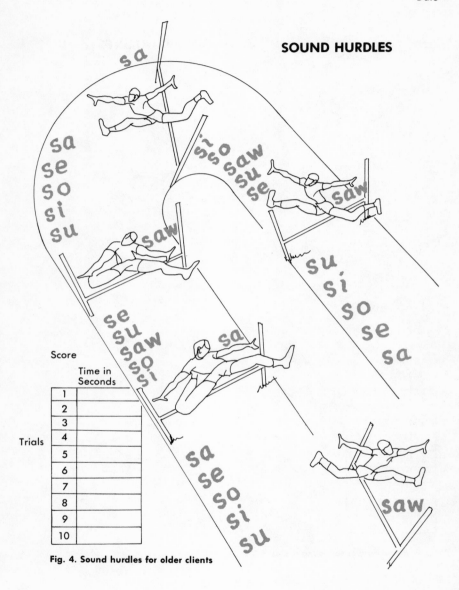

Fig. 4. Sound hurdles for older clients

elicit many repetitions of correct production, thus reinforcing the newly learned neuromuscular patterns without any accompanying boredom and fatigue.

The rhythms are determined by musical notation: the half (♩) or quarter notes (♩) indicate the longer stressed syllables; the eighth (♪) or sixteenth notes (♪) represent the short unstressed syllables (fig. 5).

Procedures

1. The clinician writes the syllables on the lines over the notes and produces the model pattern for the client. The client imitates the clinician, and may initially produce the patterns in unison with the clinician.

2. When familiar with the patterns, the client practices until production within the rhythms is fluent and consistently correct.

3. The client may compose original melodies for the rhythms and sing his syllable drills.

4. Tape-record the rhythm drills, particularly evaluating the unstressed syllables for correct sound production.

Model Sentences

Practicing syllables in the rhythm and melody patterns of spontaneous speech is one more step toward the incorporation of the corrected sound into conversation. Each sentence presents a different stress pattern, the underlined word in the model indicating where the primary stress should be placed.

Stimulus Materials

1. During initial attempts, each line of squares may be composed of the same repeated syllable (fig. 6, left-hand examples).

2. Later practice may be made more challenging by using different syllables in all the squares in one row (fig. 6, right-hand examples).

3. The rhythm blocks are readily adaptable to drill with variations of syllables to serve the needs of individual cases: initial and final blends (fig. 7, upper examples); drills for reinforcement of tongue-alveolar ridge placement in correction of tongue thrust (fig. 7, lower examples).

Procedures

1. The clinician reads the model sentence, emphasizing the stress pattern by tapping the table or by clapping hands.

FOLLOW THE BEAT

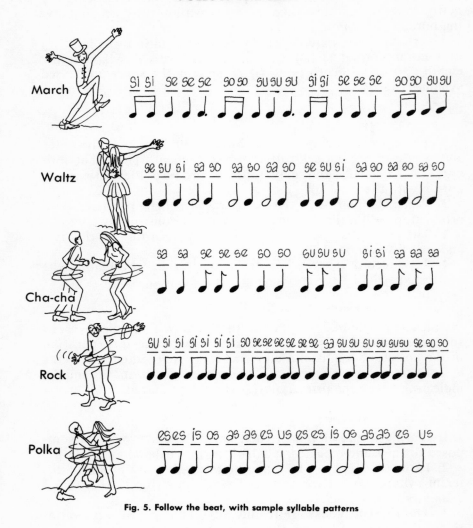

Fig. 5. Follow the beat, with sample syllable patterns

MODEL SENTENCE DRILLS

Practice syllables in the rhythm of the model sentences.
Work toward the speed of conversational speech.

<u>Where</u> is my coat?

sa	sa	sa	sa
se	se	se	se
si	si	si	si
so	so	so	so
su	su	su	su

Oh, <u>here</u> it is.

sa	so	se	si
se	si	su	sa
si	su	se	so
so	sa	si	se
su	se	so	si

I can't <u>hear</u> you.

ās	as	as	as
ēs	es	es	es
īs	is	is	is
ōs	os	os	os
ūs	us	us	us

Will you come <u>here</u>?

as	es	os	is
es	us	as	os
is	as	us	es
os	es	is	as
us	is	as	os

Fig. 6. Model sentences with different stress patterns. The examples in the left-hand boxes show repetition of the same syllables for initial attempts; the right-hand boxes use different syllables in each square per row.

MODEL SENTENCE DRILLS

Practice syllables in the rhythm of the model sentences. Work toward the speed of conversational speech.

Where is my coat?

sta	sta	sta	sta
ske	ske	ske	ske
smi	smi	smi	smi
slo	slo	slo	slo
snu	snu	snu	snu

Oh, here it is.

ăst	ast	ast	ast
ěst	est	est	est
ĭst	íst	íst	íst
ŏst	ost	ost	ost
ŭst	ust	ust	ust

I can't hear you.

ats	ats	ats	ats
ets	ets	ets	ets
its	its	íts	its
ots	ots	ots	ots
uts	uts	uts	uts

Will you come here?

ans	ans	ans	ans
its	its	its	íts
eds	eds	eds	eds
íns	ins	íns	ins
ats	ats	ats	ats

Fig. 7. Model sentences with different stress patterns. The examples in the two upper boxes are drills with initial and final blends; those in the two lower boxes are for reinforcement of tongue-alveolar ridge placement.

2. The clinician writes appropriate syllables in the squares, saying the syllables in one row to the rhythm of the model sentence. The client imitates the model. The same procedure is used for each row of squares in one rhythm block.

3. For the next block of syllables, the same procedure is followed, but in the rhythm of *its* model sentence.

4. All the syllable stress patterns are practiced until they can be produced at the speed and in the rhythm of running speech.

5. For the development of self-monitoring skills, the client is asked to evaluate his production at the end of each row. He is required to state whether all syllables were produced correctly. Errors must be identified by number; he must say that, for example, syllables two and three were not correct. In this way, he develops pinpoint precision in self-evaluation.

NONSENSE WORDS

Stimulus Materials

The nonsense word can be a potent therapeutic tool if it is used prescriptively. Each client's difficulty in configurational productions should be analyzed and used as a basis for the construction of pseudowords tailor-made for his needs. For example, if a client cannot produce an [s] within a word when it precedes or follows a stop-plosive, these abutting consonants should be embedded into the nonsense words designed for his therapy.

Procedures

Nonsense words may be introduced in the hopscotch and practiced in the sound hurdles (figs. 8 and 9).

1. In hopscotch, follow the same procedures as for syllable hopscotch drill. At first, each word will be produced separately in imitation of the clinician. As the client gains greater familiarity with the nonsense words through practice, he can produce them in groups of two or three, on one breath, according to the block groupings in the hopscotch. Ultimately, the nine words should be produced in connected utterance on one breath.

2. Place a check in a score block each time the pattern is completed without error.

3. Procedures for practicing with nonsense words in the hurdles are the same as for syllable drill.

Enjoyable home assignments may consist of inventing original nonsense words. Subsequent activity may be the formation

SOUND HOPSCOTCH

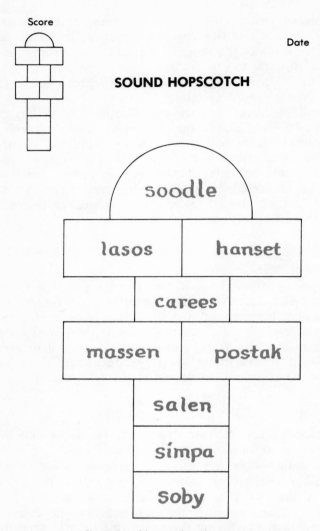

Fig. 8. Sound hopscotch with nonsense words.

SOUND HURDLES

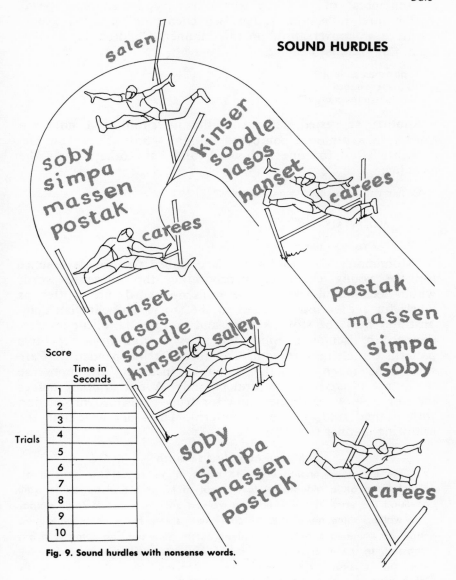

salen

kinser
soodle
lasos
hanset

carees

soby
simpa
massen
postak

carees

postak
massen
simpa
soby

hanset
lasos
soodle
kinser salen

soby
simpa
massen
postak

carees

Score

Time in
Seconds

Trials	
1	
2	
3	
4	
5	
6	
7	
8	
9	
10	

Fig. 9. Sound hurdles with nonsense words.

of "sentences" of nonsense words using conversational speed, rhythm, and inflection. Either two clients or an entire group can have a "conversation" in this manner. Children enjoy talking in this "foreign language."

"Soby massen lasos?"
"Sikesoo samosa salen carees."
"Postak simpa hanset!"

Another suggested activity is the insertion of a nonsense word into a sentence composed of real words. Substitute the nonsense word for one real word, and have others guess the meaning:

"When you leave, don't bang the soby."

MOONTALK

For Young Clients

"Moonman's Visit to Earth," is designed to provide practice for the young client in incorporating the nonsense words within meaningful speech. The nonsense words are written as labels for the various pictures in the story. The clinician demonstrates how the story is told, and at first the client imitates sentence by sentence. Since the story is told in a repetitive pattern, the clients are soon able to tell it independently. Care should be taken that the sentences including the nonsense words are uttered with natural prosody. Avoid stopping before the nonsense word; rather, aim for truly connected production with normal rate and stress patterns. The story is told in the following manner (fig. 10).

Moonman's Visit to Earth

One day a Moonman came to earth in his rocket (or spaceship). He landed on a mountain. He got out of his ship and began to walk around the earth. He walked and walked until he came to some *simpa*. He walked some more until he came to a *salen*. He walked some more until he came to a *soby*. He walked some more until he came to a big *massen*. In the *massen* he saw many *lasos*. He walked some more until he saw a *carees*. He walked some more until he saw a *sikasoo*. By that time he was so tired that he walked back to his ship and blasted off. S-s-s-s-s-s-s-s-s-s!

Children enjoy tape-recording the story and producing a satisfying facsimile of a blast-off by holding the microphone close to the mouth while they say the sound very loudly.

MOONTALK PICTURE FORM

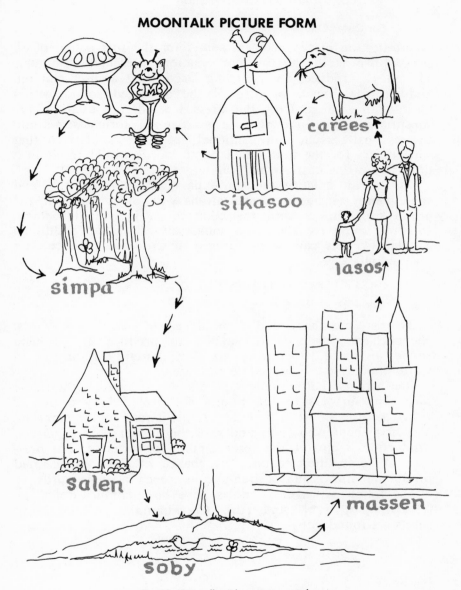

Fig. 10. Moontalk with nonsense words.

For Older Clients

Substitution of the problem sound for the first sound of all stressed words in the two conversations presented in figures 11 and 12 produces an intriguing jargon that amuses children and provides much practice of the corrected sound within meaningful context. Only the stressed words are used for the substitutions, since the purpose is to retain normal stress and unstress patterns at conversational speed. It is believed that substitution for the first sound of all words would result in a distortion of the unstress pattern.

Clients can practice the entire passages alone initially, and subsequently engage in conversations with other clients in the group situation or with the clinician in individual therapy. Children enjoy recording the conversations. As an additional assignment, they can be encouraged to write and practice their own moontalk.

PRODUCTION OF REAL WORDS

Riddles

By the time the sound is produced in meaningful words, clients have developed the ability to produce the problem sound at speed. Therefore, no slow, careful production in words should be encouraged or permitted.

One activity that stimulates production at speed is the riddle race. The answers to the riddles are provided by means of either pictures or word lists. The riddle is read by the clinician. The first client who finds and says the answer wins a point *if* production is correct. He loses a point for an error. The pressure of competition reduces the chance of slow, exaggerated production and facilitates spontaneous speech in single words.

The following rhymed riddles have been composed for [s], [r], [l], [sh], [ch], and [th]. Corresponding picture work sheets are found in figs. 13-18.

MOONTALK STORIES

Get set for blast-off.
Are all systems go?
Everything is A-O.K.
Countdown. 10-9-8-7-6-5-4-3-2-1-
Blast off!
We're in orbit.
Now we're headed for the moon.
There it is. It's coming closer.
Prepare for landing.
Landing module has separated.
We're coming in on target.
We made it! It was a perfect landing.
Look, there's someone out there.
Wow! There really is a man on the moon.
Hello, Moonman. We can talk moontalk.

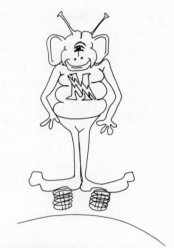

Figs. 11 and 12. Moontalk with target sound substituted for initial sound in stressed words

Substitute your sound for the sounds that are underlined.

Hello, Mickey. How are you?
I'm fine, thank you.
Listen, I'm having a costume party on Hallowe'en. Can you come?
What time will it be?
It will begin at eight o'clock.
Who else is coming?
Just come and be surprised.
It sounds like a lot of fun.
We should have a ball. A lot of the kids from school will be here.
Thanks for asking me. I'll be there! Goodbye.
Goodbye.

[s] RIDDLES

SUN	Shiny and yellow and hot and bright. We see it by day but not by night.
CROSS	One bar goes this way, and one bar goes that; sometimes you see it on a nurse's hat.
MOUSE	When he skitters and scampers around the house, we hear him squeak and know it's a _____.
BASKET	When we play a-tisket a-tasket, we say we have lost our little yellow _____
DRESS	It's something to wear and to enjoy; it's something to wear, but not for a boy.
SAW	You'll find it in a tool box—at least, you should. Its edge is jagged, and it cuts through wood.
ICE CREAM	Chocolate, vanilla, strawberry, peach. Everyone loves it; there's a flavor for each.
SEESAW	Up and down, up and down. Sometimes in the air, sometimes on the ground.
SEVEN	It comes after six; it rhymes with eleven. It comes before eight, and so of course it is _____.
SOAP	You use it on dishes, you use it on pans; you use it on face, you use it on hands.
SAUCER	There's many a slip 'twixt the cup and the lip. What do you see that catches the drip?
HOUSE	It has four walls, a roof, and a floor. It has many windows and a door.
SAILBOAT	Blow, wind, blow. Make it go.
BUS	When we go to school, it comes for us. We all like to ride on the big orange _____.
BRACELET	Sometimes it's silver, sometimes it's gold; sometimes it's new, sometimes it's old.
SEAL	It barks like a dog and swims like a fish; and fish is really its favorite dish.

[s] RIDDLES

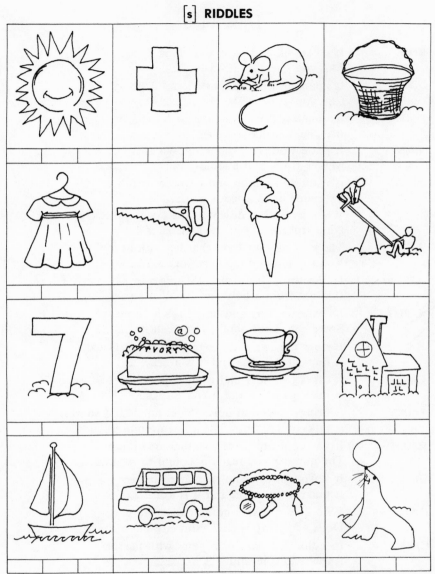

Fig. 13. [s]-riddle pictures

[r] RIDDLES

RING	It's a round and hard and shiny thing; Can you guess it? It's a _____.
DOOR	It's part of a house, but it's not a floor; Can you guess it? It's a _____.
TURTLE	Its name is Pokey or Sam or Myrtle; It's slow and hard-shelled, and it is a _____.
RAIN	It patters on roof and window pane; Makes rivers and puddles, and it is _____.
BEAR	It's soft and plump and covered with hair; Everyone loves a teddy _____.
RAKE	When leaves fall down on the lawn and make An awful mess, you use a _____.
EAR	The part of your head that lets you hear, You surely know is called an _____.
ARROW	It flies through the air. It's long and narrow; It's shot from a bow and is called an _____.
RABBIT	Its ears are long and hopping's a habit; Some call it cottontail, some call it _____.
BIRD	It sings the sweetest songs you've ever heard; It hops and it flies and it is a _____.
CAR	It takes you near and it takes you far; It takes gasoline and it is a _____.
RADIO	It brings news and music from north and south; It talks and it sings, but it has no mouth.
FOUR	If you count to three and then one more, The number you reach is bound to be _____.
FIRE	It starts out low and then leaps higher; It makes you warm and it is a _____.
GIRL	Who likes dresses and hair that will curl; Dolls and jump ropes? Who else but a _____.
CARROT	Its color is orange; it rhymes with parrot; Rabbits love it, and it is a _____.

[r] RIDDLES

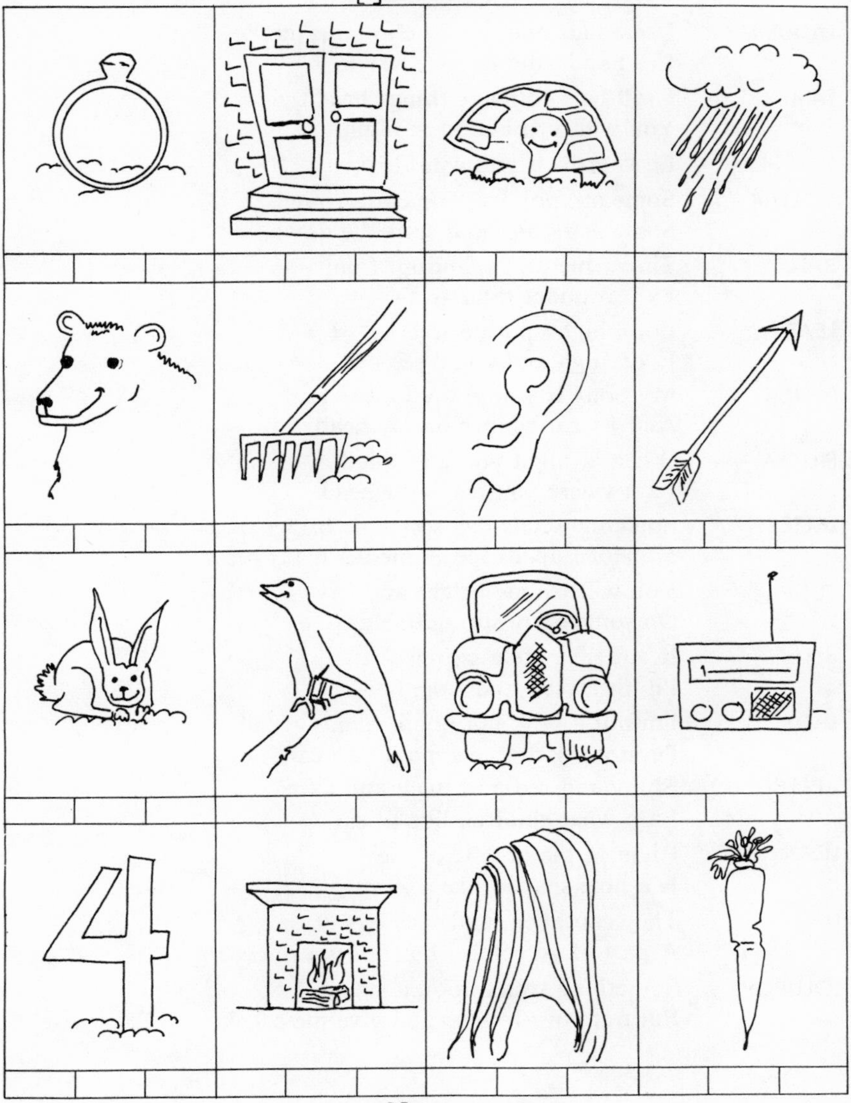

Fig. 14. [r]-riddle pictures

[l] RIDDLES

LADDER	Use hands and feet to climb up me; Use hands and feet so carefully.
LAMP	I will help to make things bright; You will turn me on at night.
BALLOON	I can grow if you will blow.
COLLAR	Some are pointed, some are round; Some stand up, and some lie down.
BALL	Throw me down, and up I go; I am rounder than an O.
LEAF	Look high up on a tree; Look high and you'll see me.
PENCIL	My body is wood, my foot is lead; And I wear rubber on my head.
PILLOW	When at night you go to bed, I am where you rest your head.
LETTER	Someone sends me, someone brings me; Someone opens me, someone reads me.
TULIP	You will see me bright and gay On some early springtime day.
BELL	If you give me a swing, I'll hit myself and ring.
LADY	I'm not a boy. I'm not a man. I'm not a girl: guess me if you can.
APPLE	Shiny and red and juicy and sweet, I am what children like to eat.
LOCK	Right in the middle of me Is a hole shaped like a key.
LIPS	They can open, and they can close; A part of your face, but not your nose.
LOLLIPOP	Something sweet upon a stick; Put out your tongue and give me a lick.

[I] RIDDLES

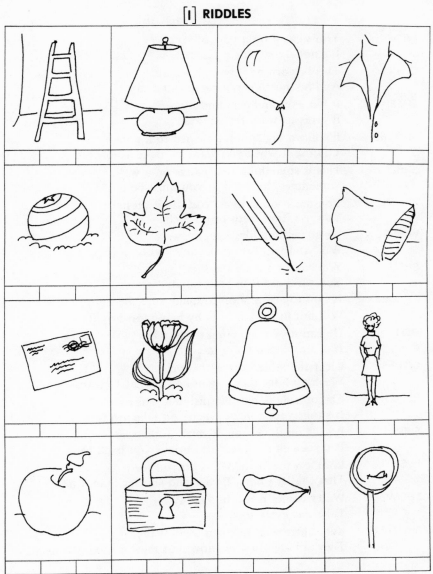

Fig. 15. [I]-riddle pictures

[sh] RIDDLES

SHOE   You wear it on a part of you;
            It's not a coat; it's a _____

SHIRT   This is worn by a boy or a man,
            And he must keep it clean as he can.

SHEEP   It has eyes and ears and a nose;
            It gives us wool for clothes.

SHOVEL   It's like a big spoon attached to a pole;
            You use it when you want to make a hole.

SHELF   This is something that hangs on a wall;
            Sometimes, to reach it, you must be tall.

BRUSH   You use it on clothes; you use it on hair;
            You use it on teeth or on a chair.

WISHBONE   It's something like a tug-of-war;
            Win, and you get what you're wishing for.

SHELL   You can find it on the sand;
            You can hold it in your hand.

SHADE   It's on top of a lamp to make sure the light
            Will not hurt your eyes by being too bright.

FISH   He can move but cannot walk;
            Has a mouth but doesn't talk.

DISHES   Clear the table, scrape them clean;
            Wash and dry them—you know what I mean.

RADISH   The outside is red; the inside is white;
            It stings your tongue when you take a bite.

SHIP   It sails on the ocean; it sails on the sea;
            It takes you far away and brings you back to me.

BUSH   Look on the lawn. What do you see
            That's taller than a flower and shorter than a tree?

SHOWER   Water comes down in a spray;
            Take one every day.

SHUTTERS   Keep them shut or open them wide;
            They're hung on a window, but they're usually outside.

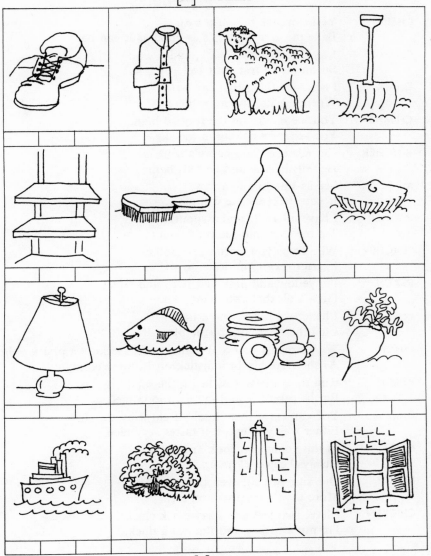

Fig. 16. [sh]-riddle pictures

[ch] RIDDLES

CHERRY
You can pick me off a tree.
Bake me in a pie that's as good as it can be.

CHAIR
I have four legs, a back, and a seat.
Sit on me to rest your feet.

CHALK
I am something that can write.
When I write, I write white.

CHIMNEY
You see me up on the roof so high.
You see me smoking in the sky.

BUTCHER
He sells beef, and he sells lamb
He sells bacon, and he sells ham.

MATCHES
See us standing in a row.
If you strike us, we will glow.

PITCHER
I have a handle and a spout.
Tip me over and the water pours out.

TEACHER
Who helps you learn to be polite,
Learn to read and learn to write?

PEACH
I'm yellow and pink and juicy and sweet
I'm a fruit that you like to eat.

WATCH
I have two hands and a face.
I tell the time but not the place.

WITCH
With straggly hair and pointy nose, she's not a pretty sight
As she rides her broomstick on Hallowe'en night.

BEACH
Run from the waves, lie on the sand,
But be careful you don't get too tanned.

CHEESE
You can eat it in a chunk or eat it by the slice.
Either way you eat it, it tastes very nice.

KITCHEN
In this room you cook and eat.
Always keep it clean and neat.

BENCH
One sits; two sit; even three.
More than one can sit on me.

CHICKEN
I have two feet and I say cluck cluck.
I'm not a turkey and I'm not a duck.

[ch] RIDDLES

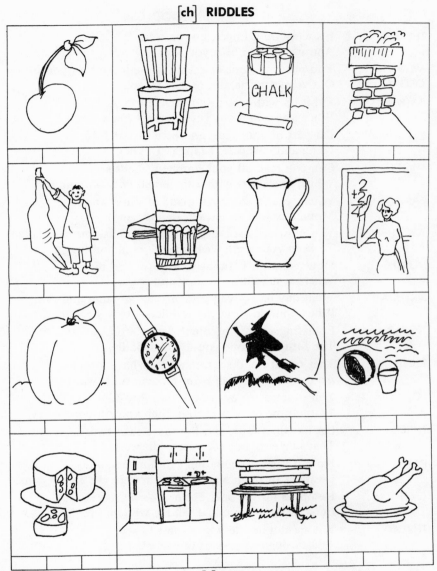

Fig. 17. [ch] -riddle pictures

[th] RIDDLES

THIMBLE	It's worn on a finger, not on a toe, And it's used to help you sew.
MOUTH ORGAN	You put it to your lips, and through the hole you blow. Out comes music, do, re, mi, fa, so.
BATHTUB	Fill it up with water and then climb in. When you climb out you'll have a clean skin.
MOUTH	I'm part of your face, and here's what I do. I sing and I whistle; I talk and I chew.
THIRTY	Can you read all your numbers? Let's see if you know Which one starts with a three and ends with an 0.
EARTH	What's round as a ball, made of water and land, Mountains and rivers, ocean and sand?
TOOTHBRUSH	You must use me every morning and use me every night To keep your teeth clean and shining and bright.
NORTH	Down south it is sunny and warm and nice. Where is it cold with snow and ice?
BIRTHDAY	What day brings you presents and goodies and fun, When you blow out the candles—every single one?
THUMB	Four fingers are "pointer," "ring," "pinky," and "middle." The fifth is the one you use to twiddle.
TEETH	They're hard and sharp, and they have a bite, And you must brush them to keep them white.
TOOTHPASTE	You squeeze me out of a tube every day. You put me in your mouth, then you rinse me away.
THREE	I'm less than four, and I'm more than two. That's an easy one for you to do.
PATH	I'm not very straight, and I'm not very wide. I wander through a garden or through the countryside.
THIEF	He opens up the safe, but he doesn't have a key. Look at the picture and tell me who you see.
THREAD	You need a needle if you want to sew, And through the eye of the needle I go.

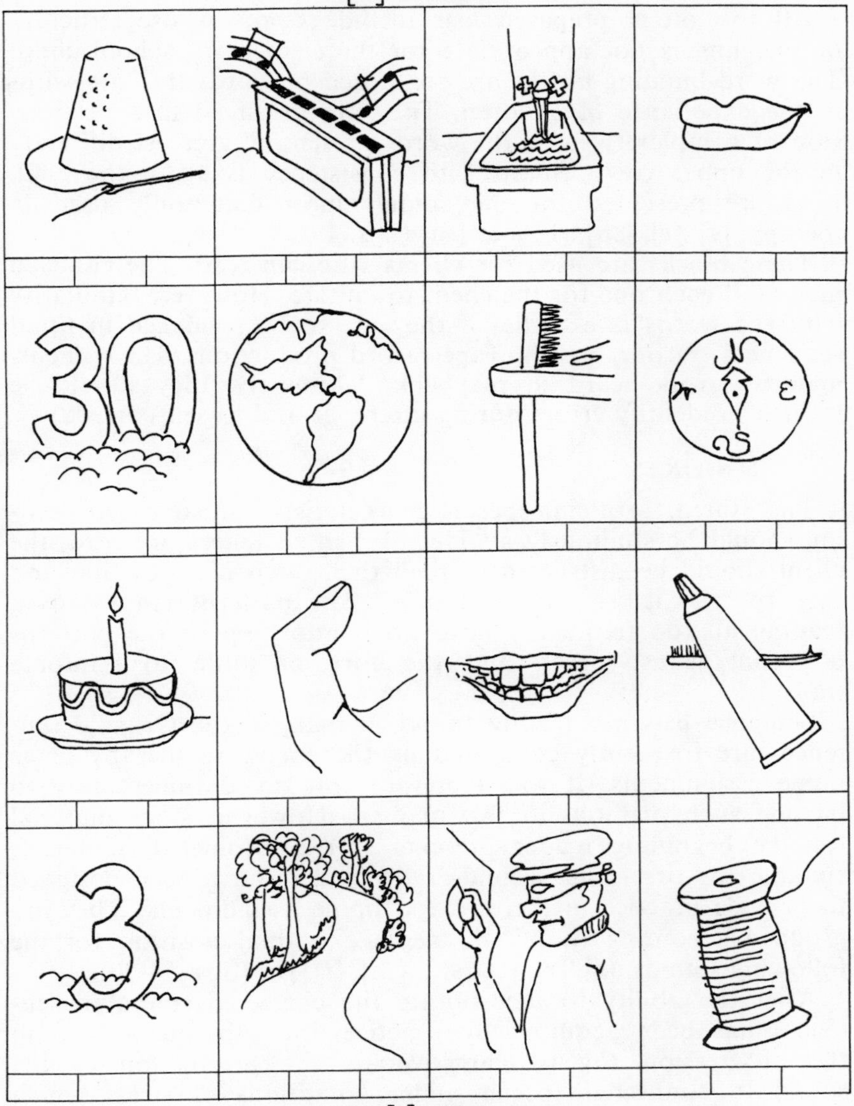

Fig. 18. [th] -riddle pictures

Word-Building Blocks

All too often, prepared lists include words whose structure or meaning is not appropriate for the elementary school child. The word-building blocks are composed of words that are within the experience of children. They are arranged in a progression of complexity, with the words presenting greatest difficulty in the upper rows. Speed with consistency is again the goal. Lists are presented for the sounds most commonly used in therapy: [s], [r], [sh], [l], and [th] (figs. 19-23).

These blocks are used for clients who can read. The clinician may read each one for the client to imitate. However, familiarity with the words is essential if they are to be produced in rapid sequences on one breath. Tape-record productions. Have clients identify errors heard in playback. Ultimately, they should be trained to identify errors during utterance and to self-correct.

SENTENCES

The stilted, artificial speech characteristic of so much reading should be studiously avoided. When sentences are read, the client should be instructed to read them with his eyes first and then to "say it the way you talk." The patterns employed in reading all too frequently have no relationship to the patterns of spontaneous speech and therefore do little to reinforce transfer.

Sentence lists are readily found in many texts. Original sentences are frequently composed by the clients in therapy or as home assignments. It was therefore considered unnecessary to include such material in this manual. However, since material for the beginning reader presents special problems, sentences suitable for first- and second-grade readers have been designed to provide practice in therapy and home assignments. They are grouped according to initial, medial, or final position for the following sounds: [s], [r], [l], [sh], [th], [f], [k] (figs. 24-30).

After the ability to incorporate the corrected sound in sentences has been acquired by practice, the subsequent goal in the progression toward carryover is the production of the sound in connected speech under conditions of stress which preclude careful, deliberate utterance. When attention can be focused on content without detriment to the mechanics of production, a major step has been taken toward the achievement of the automaticity characteristic of spontaneous speech.

Each of the following suggested activities is designed to elicit responses under the pressure of a time limit. Points are

[s]-SOUND WORD BLOCKS

Build the word blocks. Start at the bottom. Say each block slowly.
Then see how fast you can go with no mistakes.

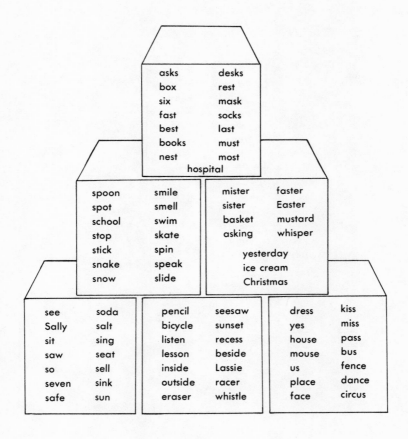

asks	desks		
box	rest		
six	mask		
fast	socks		
best	last		
books	must		
nest	most		
	hospital		

spoon	smile	mister	faster
spot	smell	sister	Easter
school	swim	basket	mustard
stop	skate	asking	whisper
stick	spin		
snake	speak	yesterday	
snow	slide	ice cream	
		Christmas	

see	soda	pencil	seesaw	dress	kiss
Sally	salt	bicycle	sunset	yes	miss
sit	sing	listen	recess	house	pass
saw	seat	lesson	beside	mouse	bus
so	sell	inside	Lassie	us	fence
seven	sink	outside	racer	place	dance
safe	sun	eraser	whistle	face	circus

Fig. 19. [s]-sound word blocks

[r]-SOUND WORD BLOCKS

Build the word blocks. Start at the bottom. Say each block slowly.
Then see how fast you can go with no mistakes.

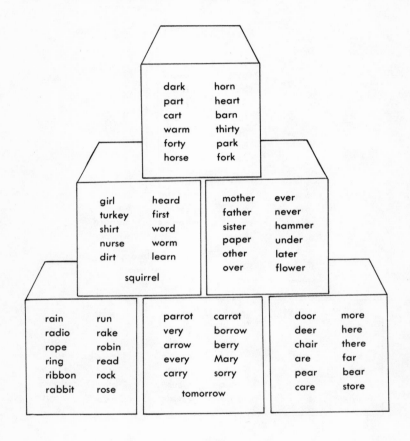

dark	horn
part	heart
cart	barn
warm	thirty
forty	park
horse	fork

girl	heard		mother	ever
turkey	first		father	never
shirt	word		sister	hammer
nurse	worm		paper	under
dirt	learn		other	later
	squirrel		over	flower

rain	run		parrot	carrot		door	more
radio	rake		very	borrow		deer	here
rope	robin		arrow	berry		chair	there
ring	read		every	Mary		are	far
ribbon	rock		carry	sorry		pear	bear
rabbit	rose			tomorrow		care	store

Fig. 20. [r]-sound word blocks

[sh]-SOUND WORD BLOCKS

Build the word blocks. Start at the bottom. Say each block slowly.
Then see how fast you can go with no mistakes.

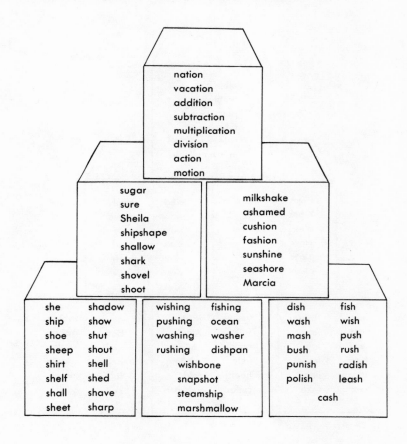

Fig. 21. [sh]-sound word blocks

[l]-SOUND WORD BLOCKS

Build the word blocks. Start at the bottom. Say each block slowly.
Then see how fast you can go with no mistakes.

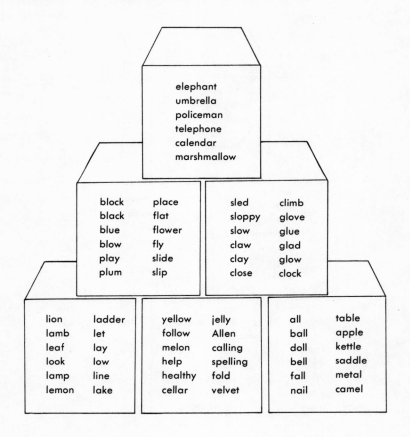

elephant	
umbrella	
policeman	
telephone	
calendar	
marshmallow	

block	place	sled	climb
black	flat	sloppy	glove
blue	flower	slow	glue
blow	fly	claw	glad
play	slide	clay	glow
plum	slip	close	clock

lion	ladder	yellow	jelly	all	table
lamb	let	follow	Allen	ball	apple
leaf	lay	melon	calling	doll	kettle
look	low	help	spelling	bell	saddle
lamp	line	healthy	fold	fall	metal
lemon	lake	cellar	velvet	nail	camel

Fig. 22. [l]-sound word blocks

[th]-SOUND WORD BLOCKS

Build the word blocks. Start at the bottom. Say each block slowly.
Then see how fast you can go with no mistakes.

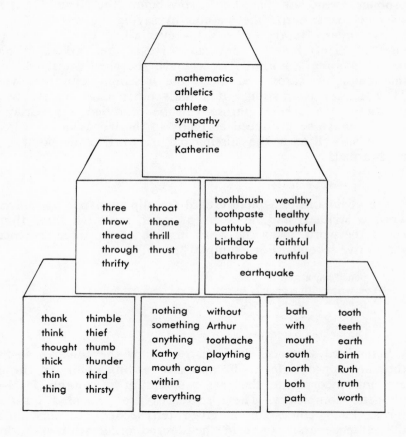

mathematics
athletics
athlete
sympathy
pathetic
Katherine

three	throat	
throw	throne	
thread	thrill	
through	thrust	
thrifty		

toothbrush	wealthy
toothpaste	healthy
bathtub	mouthful
birthday	faithful
bathrobe	truthful
earthquake	

thank	thimble
think	thief
thought	thumb
thick	thunder
thin	third
thing	thirsty

nothing	without
something	Arthur
anything	toothache
Kathy	plaything
mouth organ	
within	
everything	

bath	tooth
with	teeth
mouth	earth
south	birth
north	Ruth
both	truth
path	worth

Fig. 23. [th] -sound word blocks

awarded only when the desired response is uttered with problem sounds correctly produced.

Guessing Game

A number of picture cards depicting words containing the problem sound are placed in a row before the client. He is instructed to memorize the pictures by saying the words in order a few times. He then closes his eyes while the clinician (or another client) removes one card. He is then asked, "Which one is missing?" Within five seconds, the client must examine the remaining cards and recall the missing picture, replying, "The _____ is missing." If sounds other than [s] are being practiced, the carrier phrase can be modified appropriately. Sounds must be produced correctly in the words in the carrier phrase as well as in the missing picture word if the point is to be awarded.

Speedy Sentences

The client draws a picture card (or slip of paper on which a word is written) and, at a given signal, must tell three things about the word, using the word in each of the three sentences, within five seconds. For example, "pencil":

"A pencil has a point."
"You write with a pencil."
"A pencil is made of wood."

Scrambled Sentences

Scrambled sentences are constructed by the clinician so that they are appropriate to the age and reading ability of the client and incorporate the target sound at a suitable level of phonetic complexity. These sentences are presented on flash cards. Each contestant is given ten seconds to unscramble the sentence and say it in the desired order with all sounds produced correctly. If he fails to do this in the allotted time, the card is displayed to another contestant. A point is earned upon successful completion of both tasks. If, however, the sentence is uttered in correct sequence but the sounds are produced defectively, a point is lost. Thus, the primary emphasis on the goal of correct production is maintained, thereby avoiding the trap of much game therapy wherein involvement in the game aspect overshadows the therapeutic aims.

$15.00

GOAL: Carryover

An Articulation Manual and Program

ADELE GERBER

The stages of articulation therapy have been described as acquisition, generalization, and automatization. The literature devoted to the acquisition of target sounds is fairly extensive, but little has been published in the area of carryover—the consistent ability to use the correct sound appropriately and in all speaking situations. Here is a manual and program which provides a procedure for achieving carryover, the problem which most speech clinicians describe as presenting the greatest difficulty in articulation therapy.

Designed for that phase of training which follows the acquisition of target sound, this program proceeds step by step toward the goal of automatization. The carefully planned exercises systematically develop automatic control to the point where the child can focus his attention on the content of the message. The remarkable degree of success which the author and her colleagues have experienced with hundreds of school-age children testifies to the value of the method.

Parts I and II of the manual present materials and techniques appropriate for use with any sound. Part III is devoted to a program of [r] therapy which involves unique problems. The exercises include rhythm drills, riddles, word-games, and fill-in stories. A pocket contains 29 loose worksheets, and 36 figures in the text explain how to use these worksheets. The worksheets supplied are master copies which may be reproduced in the quantity needed for clinical use with individuals or with groups. All children may not require all included activities at all levels, but the full range of materials, systematically ordered, is provided.

Adele Gerber is Assistant Professor, Clinical Supervisor and Director of the Urban Language Institute in the Department of Speech at Temple University.

Temple University Press   •   *Philadelphia*

SENTENCES WITH [s] SOUNDS

1. I see the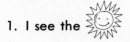

2. Dick has two

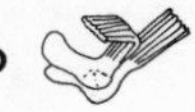

3. Look for the

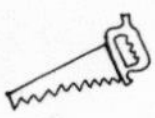

4. I like the

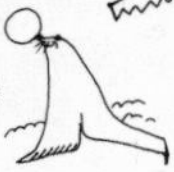

5. I ride in the

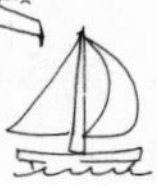

1. I like to eat

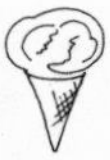

2. Play on the

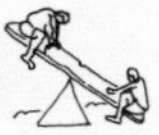

3. Put something in the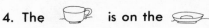

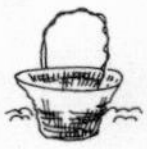

4. The 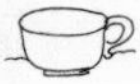 is on the

5. I ride my

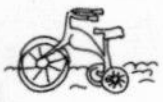

1. Come to my

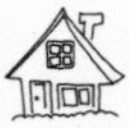

2. Sally has a blue

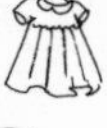

3. See the little

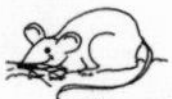

4. I have a big

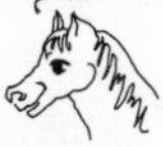

5. I ride on a

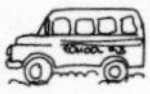

Fig. 24. Sentences with [s] sounds

SENTENCES WITH [r] SOUNDS

1. Sue has a pretty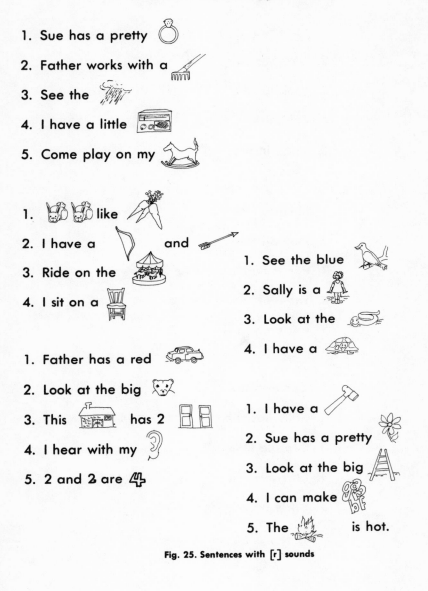
2. Father works with a
3. See the
4. I have a little
5. Come play on my

1. like
2. I have a and
3. Ride on the
4. I sit on a

1. See the blue
2. Sally is a
3. Look at the
4. I have a

1. Father has a red
2. Look at the big
3. This has 2
4. I hear with my
5. 2 and 2 are 4

1. I have a
2. Sue has a pretty
3. Look at the big
4. I can make
5. The is hot.

Fig. 25. Sentences with [r] sounds

SENTENCES WITH [ɪ] SOUNDS

1. I walk on my

2. You have red

3. Cut the

4. Mother is a

1. Sleep on a

2. My dress has a

3. He has a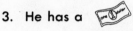

4. Talk on the

1. Catch the

2. Ring the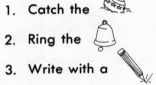

3. Write with a

4. Dig with a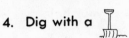

Fig. 26. Sentences with [ɪ] sounds

SENTENCES WITH [sh] SOUNDS

1. I have new

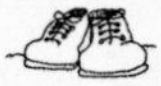

2. The 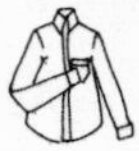 is blue.

3. He has a little

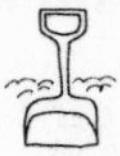

4. We sail on a big

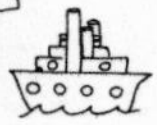

5. See my

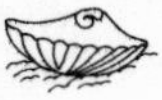

1. He is

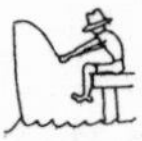

2. The 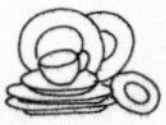 are dirty.

3. I have a

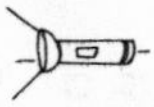

4. Jane has 2

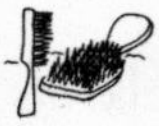

5. He broke the

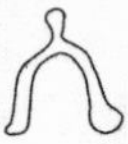

1. The 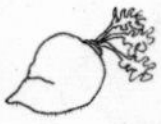 is red.

2. The 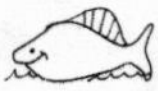 is in the water.

3. 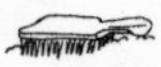 your hair.

4. The 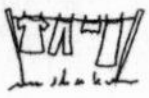 is clean.

5. See that big

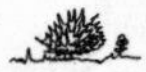

Fig. 27. Sentences with [sh] sounds

SENTENCES WITH [th] SOUNDS

1. See my

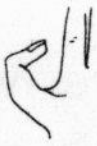

2. Count 1, 2....3

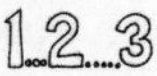

3. Mother has a

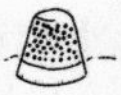

4. This book is

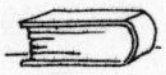

5. This book is

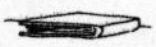

1. Happy

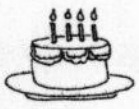

2. Go in the

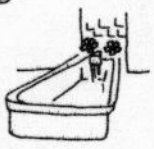

3. See my new

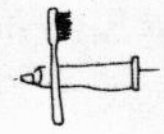

1. Look at my

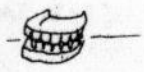

2. I lost a

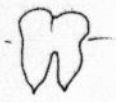

3. My 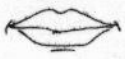 is red.

Fig. 28. Sentences with [th] sounds

1. I have two
2. Father made a
3. Father made a funny
4. The ___ is little.
5. I have five

1. Mother likes
2. I like
3. Sit on the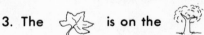

1. I cut with a
2. The ___ is on the
3. The ___ is on the
4. Get me a ___ of bread.
5. This is an Indian

Fig. 29. Sentences with [f] sounds

SENTENCES WITH [k] SOUNDS

1. Come in the 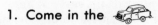.
2. I like 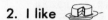.
3. Mother makes 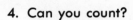.
4. Can you count?
5. The 🐱 is black.

1. Look at the 🦃.
2. Put something in my 👕.
3. I like 🦃.

1. See the 🦆 walk.
2. Dick sat on a 🏔.
3. I have a ➶.
4. My coat is on the 🪝.

Fig. 30. Sentences with [k] sounds

FILL-IN STORIES

This material has been designed to serve a number of purposes. It can be employed in early stages of therapy in ear-training activities. Subsequently, it can be used to elicit single words in a meaningful context. Finally, it can be used as a reading passage of connected speech. All of the words are found on the Bryngelson-Glaspey Picture Cards. (See figs. 31-33.)

Discrimination Activity

The pictures of words used in the story are spread before the client as the clinician reads the story. If an error is made by the clinician on a problem sound, the client turns the picture face down.

Word Production

Picture words are spread before the client. The clinician reads the story, omitting the fill-in words. The client must find and say the correct word. If he produces the sound correctly, he keeps the picture.

Pre-Carryover Story

The client fills in the blank spaces with words chosen from the lists at the bottom of the page. He then reads the entire story, producing all problem sounds correctly.

SOME CARRYOVER SUGGESTIONS

Many other sources provide material traditionally used in carryover activities: poems, skits, topics for reports, or spontaneous discussion.

I believe that an inexhaustible supply of material can be derived from the school curriculum. The use of correct production in subject matter that is a part of the daily activity outside the therapy room tends to foster transfer of learning to real-life situations. Once again, automaticity of production under conditions wherein attention must be focused on content is the ultimate goal.

Suggested Activities

Arithmetic. Have flash cards of number combinations produced with speed. Use multiplication tables. Explain orally the steps of a demonstrated problem.

FILL-IN STORIES WITH [s]-SOUND WORDS

One icy winter day, Mother asked Sue and Sam to go to the _____ .
"Take a _____ and write down the list. I need some _____ ,
some _____ , and some _____ ." Sam took his _____ ,
and Sue wore her _____ _____ . They had to _____
at the corner. A _____ was directing traffic. When they reached
the store, they asked for the _____ , the _____ , and the
_____ . They put them in the _____ and put the
_____ on the _____ . When they got home, they were so cold
they were glad to get in the _____ .

pencil   stop   policeman   basket

store   soap   strawberries   soup

sled   ice   house   skates

Fig. 31. Fill-in stories with [s]-sound words

FILL-IN STORIES WITH [r]-SOUND WORDS

One day a _____ came to a farm looking for _____ .

First, he heard a _____ coming down the _____ .

He ran to hide. Next, it began to _____ .

He ran into a _____ . There were some _____

in the barn. They started to chirp. Next he head a _____

crowing. Then he heard someone banging a _____ . It was too noisy

for the _____ . He ran out into the _____ saying,

"I'd rather be wet than deaf."

rabbit	car	robins
hammer	rain	rooster
carrots	barn	road

Fig. 32. Fill-in stories with [r]-sound words

FILL-IN STORIES WITH [sh]-SOUND WORDS

Sherman had a very busy day. First he had to tend to the _____ .

Next he took a can of paint and a _____ and painted the toolshed. Then

he went _____ . He caught quite a few _____ . He saw a big

_____ sailing in the ocean. When he came home, his _____

was a mess. His mother threw it right in the _____ _____ .

sheep	brush	ship
fishing	fish	shirt
washing	machine	

Fig. 33. Fill-in stories with [sh]-sound words

Spelling. Have clients ask each other to spell words assigned in the week's spelling list. Demonstrate how words are syllabified. Explain rules of spelling: vowel digraphs, doubled consonants, and so on.

Content subjects. Explain a science experiment that was conducted in class. Answer questions about the current social studies unit. Explain and give examples of terms in grammar and usage.

The above suggestions are intended merely to stimulate the creative imagination of the clinician. They do not exhaust the possibilities provided by the client's school experience.

Even with the best planning and therapy, transfer will not readily occur if all effort is confined to the therapy session. It is necessary to extend the awareness of the correction to actual real-life situations. In other terms, it is necessary to create discriminative stimuli outside the therapy room. A visit to the classroom teacher, with the purpose of demonstrating the corrected production to a significant person not involved in therapy, can provide impetus to the carryover process. The teacher, who has contact with the child five days a week, can serve as an enlightened monitor. All teachers I have encountered have been willing to keep a log of the child's progress in the use of the corrected sound in specified situations in the classroom. The child's awareness that the teacher is listening intensifies his own monitoring during utterance.

Parents also have been eager to assist in the same manner, by monitoring the child's attempts to incorporate the corrected sound in designated conversational situations in the home.

Samples of both the teachers' and the parents' log sheets are shown in figs. 34 and 35.

TEACHERS' LOG SHEET

To the teacher:

This child has learned to produce the _____ sound correctly. Will you please assist us in our attempts to incorporate the corrected sound into the child's connected speech pattern?

Below is a daily log on different levels of speech performance:

a. *Oral Reading*—during the regular scheduled reading period.
b. *Good Talking Time*—some specific speech situation, such as show and tell, oral report, current events, poetry recitation, etc. during which time the child will consciously try to remember to use the correct production of the sound in whatever is said. (It would be helpful if, during both of the above situations, you used a signal, pre-arranged with the child, to notify him of errors which may then be corrected unobtrusively.)
c. *Spontaneous Conversation*—your evaluation of the consistency of correct production during some period of conversation other than the good talking time, when the child is unaware of your listening check.

Indicate successful performance by "yes", lack of success by "no", and degrees of partial success by the following code:

3—correct most, but not all, of the time
2—about equal degrees of success and error
1—more errors than correct production

Thank you so much for your cooperation. I hope that our united efforts will speed this child on the way toward full correction.

Sincerely,

Speech Clinician

	Oral Reading			Good Talking Time			Spontan. Conversation		
Monday									
Tuesday									
Wednesday									
Thursday									
Friday									

Fig. 34. Teachers' log sheet

PARENTS' LOG SHEET

Dear parent:

Will you please assist us in our attempts to incorporate the correct production of your child's speech sound into the conversational speech pattern?

Below is a daily log on different levels of speech performance:

a. *Single Item Assignment*—the child is to use the corrected sound in one sentence of conversation.

b. *Good Talking Time*—the child will attempt to remember to use the correct production in whatever conversation takes place during a specific, scheduled period of time each day (approximately ¼ hour).

c. *Unscheduled Observation*—your evaluation of the consistency of correct production in spontaneous conversation during some period of conversation other than the good talking time, when the child is unaware of your listening check.

Indicate successful performance by "yes", lack of success by "no", and degrees of partial success by the following code:

3—correct most, but not all, of the time
2—about equal degrees of success and error
1—more errors than correct production

Please limit correction of the child's errors to the good talking time. A small reward at the end of the week for sincere effort and improvement might provide the incentive to motivate the child toward greater achievement.

Thank you for your cooperation.

Sincerely,

Speech Clinician

	Single Item			Good Talking Time			Unscheduled Observat'n		
Sunday									
Monday									
Tuesday									
Wednesday									
Thursday									
Friday									
Saturday									

Fig. 35. Parents' log sheet

III

AN APPROACH TO [r] CORRECTION

5

RATIONALE

THE achievement of [r] correction is recognized as one of the most difficult tasks in articulation therapy. It would appear that the [r] phoneme is different in some important ways from other commonly misarticulated consonant sounds. Probably the major difference lies in the fact that [r] is not a true consonant at all. The study by Curtis and Hardy (1959) strongly suggests that certain [r] occurrences may be more appropriately classified as vocalic sounds. In most consonant sounds, articulators provide feedback cues of touch and position. However, in vocalic sounds, wherein articulators are not brought into approximation, tongue action and position are not readily identifiable. Therefore, according to Judson and Weaver (1942), most of the control of tongue action is due primarily to auditory feedback and only secondarily to proprioceptive cues. The reduced level of tactile and kinesthetic cues does seem to contribute to the difficulty so frequently experienced in the acquisition and stabilization of the [r] allophones.

Further complicating the task of correction is the fact that the [r] phoneme includes at least six allophones. Some of these seem to function as steady-state vowels, others as consonant glides, and still others as the off-glide in diphthongs. The results of the Curtis and Hardy study revealed characteristic response patterns among different consonant [r]'s, among certain sub-classes of vowel [r]'s, and in different phonetic contexts. Clinical experience presents additional evidence that different clients may demonstrate distinctly different patterns consisting of errors on some allophones but not on others. It is considered imperative that these patterns be precisely analyzed, so that therapy time and effort may be devoted only to those allophones requiring correction and not expended on others which may be in the client's repertoire. In the present program, practice material is organized in discrete categories to promote separate mastery of each of the six allophones: prevocalic single glide, prevocalic blend, stressed syllabic, unstressed syllabic, postvocalic final, and postvocalic preconsonantal [r].

6

PRINCIPLES AND PROCEDURES
FOR ACQUISITION

ALTHOUGH the major emphasis in this manual is on the postacquisition phase of training, the unique difficulty experienced by many clinicians with the achievement of [r] production would seem to justify the sharing of any information that might facilitate acquisition. No claim for infallibility is intended. What is effective for certain clinicians with certain clients will not prove equally successful in other circumstances. However, some clinical principles have emerged from extensive work in [r] therapy that may prove helpful when applied to the management of these problems.

Of primary importance is the clinician's competence in careful analysis of the nature of the error sound and the way in which it differs from correct production. Only as a result of such analysis can the clinician tailor therapy to the individual case. Three aspects of production most generally require attention, to varying degrees and in varying combinations, in order to achieve the desired [r] quality: tongue elevation, tension, and/or widening.

It is widely recognized that some portion of the tongue must be raised to achieve [r] production. Although the acoustic quality can result from humping of the dorsum or retraction of the tip as well as from elevation and retroflexion of the tip and blade, the latter appears to be the easier method to teach. It should be clearly understood, however, that whenever the auditory characteristics are achieved by whatever means, tongue position is no longer the concern of the clinician.

Inspection and analysis of error production in many cases have revealed a high incidence of a few frequently occurring patterns. The first commonly observed activity is a shift of tension from the tongue to the lips, which assume a rounded position closely resembling the one used in producing a [w]. Another pattern involves displacement of tension from the tongue to the lower jaw and lip, often in conjunction with elevation of those structures. The latter aspect may be regarded as displacement of elevation from the tongue to the mandible, the former remaining low in the mouth and relatively inert.

There are times during therapy when tongue elevation is achieved without production of [r] quality. Closer examination of this phenomenon will usually reveal either inadequate tension in the musculature or a narrowing and pointing of the tongue.

Procedures have been developed to aid in solving these problems. Although these procedures are effective, results are seldom instantaneous. The identification and disruption of subtle, well-established neuromotor patterns require time, and the substitution of new patterns, calling for refined and complex coordination and control, takes even more time. However, the elimination of patterns that interfere with the achievement of target production is usually accomplished by specific remediating cues more readily than by the general exhortation, "Try it again."

Use of the mirror, in which the client's and clinician's faces are in close approximation, is helpful in directing attention to crucial actions of tongue, lips, and jaw. Demonstration and imitation are preferable to explication. When verbal cues are necessary, vivid verbal imagery has been found effective in achieving desired placement indirectly. Examples will be given below in connection with other techniques. Modification of other sounds is preferable to direct phonetic placement.

Whenever possible, the simplest, least involved approach should be taken first. Integral stimulation (Milisen 1954), by means of clear, forceful auditory and visual cues presented without verbal explication is preferable. To ensure effectiveness, the clinician must so structure the demonstration that the visual as well as the auditory cues are highly evident.

If attention is to be drawn to tongue action, the clinician must be sufficiently self-aware to maintain adequate opening between upper and lower jaws to permit observation. If the client is to attempt to imitate the model and monitor his imitation he must be able to see both himself and the model in the mirror. Too often, the clinician sees his own and the client's images and is not sufficiently attuned to the client's situation to check his access to the reflected faces.

Sometimes merely presenting a sustained [ɝ] repeatedly, shaping the client's approximations toward the target by selective reinforcement is an effective approach. However, when little change over many trials is evident, it is frequently helpful to demonstrate tongue action from a low vowel, such as [ɑ], or a front vowel, such as [e], to the [ɝ] position. Here, kinesthetic cues are added to the visual and auditory cues. I have found that movement from [ɑ] or [e] to the prolonged [ɝ] and back to the vowel is frequently successful in mobilizing an inert tongue. If necessary verbal cues may be added to focus attention on tongue, lips, and jaw action.

In cases where the tongue is narrowed, making no contact at the lateral margins with the upper molars, a switch to [i] can be effective—that is, [iɝi]—by automatically widening the tongue. In such cases, with young clients in particular, I have resorted to verbal cues such as, "Keep your train (the tongue) on both tracks (contact with molars) and slide it back into the tunnel (retract the tongue)."

There are cases where none of the above methods have produced the desired results, and more deliberately controlled phonetic placement appears to be necessary.

One such approach that has proved highly successful in most cases was designed to provide a tactile frame of reference within which the tongue can orient itself. As was stated above, since [r] is predominantly vowel-like, its production involves few perceptible articulatory contacts. The technique described below guides the tongue, in a tracking procedure, by means of a set of discernible cues to the target position.

Demonstrate the following steps, which the client is to imitate.

1. Start with a voiced th, [ð], having the client match position by looking in the mirror beside you. Maintain continuous vocalization, the vibrations of which will heighten awareness of tongue contacts.

2. *Very slowly*, retract the tongue so that it maintains constant contact with a series of oral structures by moving up the back of the upper incisors, across the alveolar ridge to the point

where it barely loses contact. Verbal instructions can be provided, as follows: "I am going to make a tongue sound [ð]. Watch as I slowly pull my tongue inside my mouth and up the back wall of my top teeth, across the bumpy road until I come to my growl spot. I will go very slowly, so that I always know exactly where my tongue is and where it is going. My motor will keep running. When I hear the growl sound, I will keep my tongue in that spot. Now, you copy me and do exactly what I did."

3. Should the client's tongue point and become narrow, he can be told to look in the mirror and "see the piece of baloney in my sandwich" (tongue spread wide between upper and lower teeth). The point is stressed that the tongue is not a hot dog (narrowed, pointed).

Extreme slowness is required in the tracking procedure in order to monitor the tongue's action. Intensive concentration on visual cues from the mirror is indispensable in early efforts. At times, if necessary, the distraction of voicing can be eliminated for a period of time in order to focus complete attention on the specific attributes of the neuromotor act and to intensify awareness of the proprioceptive cues.

If the lips tend to round or if the bottom lip elevates, achieve the necessary retraction or lowering indirectly by focusing attention on the number of upper and lower teeth that should be visible. By concentrating on the exposure of four top and four bottom teeth, the lips retract subvolitionally.

Eventually, the prolonged "growl" can be segmented into a series of shorter vocalic [ɝ]'s. When these have been stabilized to the point where they can be achieved without movement from the interdental position, the vocalic or syllabic [ɝ] is ready for stabilization in combination with vowels and/or consonants in syllables.

On occasion, although position has been achieved, it appears that there is insufficient muscle tone in the tongue to produce strong [r] coloration. In such cases, any or all of the following suggestions may prove helpful.

Rapidly wiggle, in fishlike fashion, the elevated tongue from side to side across the "growl spot." This action seems to increase muscle tone and produce the desired resonance.

Press the client's thumb under your chin at about the point where the tongue muscles are inserted. Start phonating [ʌ], then glide to [ɝ], demonstrating an increase in muscle tension perceptible to the touch. Have the client repeat the action with his thumb under his own chin.

If all else fails, resistance therapy can sometimes be employed by having the client press a tongue depressor against the underside of your tongue. You can demonstrate that during [r]-less production of the central vowel the tongue is like a "pillow" and can be easily pushed around. When you shift to the [r]-colored vowel, the tongue becomes like a "board," thus demonstrating the increase in muscle tone. The client can then repeat this action against his own tongue to achieve the desired tension.

Once the vocalic [ɝ] has been achieved, its stabilization depends largely on auditory cues, since the unenhanced tactile and kinesthetic cues do not lend themselves so readily to monitoring. When this vocalic [ɝ] can be produced in isolation approximately 75 percent of the time, I would consider acquisition accomplished. From that point, the stressed vocalic [ɝ] is used as a base from which the other allophones are developed. The balance of the present program is devoted to the progress from postacquisition to carryover.

7

PRINCIPLES AND PROCEDURES
FOR STABILIZATION

T HE structured material in this program was designed for the postacquisition phase of therapy. However, the achievement of [r] production by no means guarantees its consistency. Most clinicians are all too familiar with the elusive character of newly acquired [r] quality. Therefore, the early levels of the programmed activity are intended to facilitate stabilization of the [r] allophones, a process that usually requires a sizable amount of time and energy.

TRAINING IN SELF-MONITORING

Throughout all levels, emphasis on self-monitoring equals emphasis on production. Carrell (1968) maintains that faulty learning and habituation result in a defective feedback which causes input-output circuits to accept a misarticulation as correct. Studies by Aungst and Frick (1964), Arnold (1956), and Aufricht (1960) have drawn attention to the fact that, while discrimination of errors in the utterance of another speaker is not significantly related to articulatory proficiency, the ability to correctly evaluate one's own errors is positively related to the speaker's articulation of those sounds. In the self-monitoring of [r] production, the motor aspect is apparently subject to the command of audition. Systematic perceptual training is necessary to develop a more effective internal comparator, so that detection of the error signal may serve as a control for production. According to Van Riper and Irwin (1958), simultaneous auditory feedback is a mechanism whose development is related to effective scanning of speech output.

Arnold (1956) observes that listening to oneself on a tape recorder facilitates self-correction, since the voice, being airborne, is heard in the same manner as the voice of another speaker. Attention to self-listening under these conditions may be intensified by virtue of the elimination of the distraction of the motor activity of speech.

Based upon all the above considerations, a sequence of activities has been devised to develop the intensified simultaneous auditory feedback necessary to the monitoring of [r] production. These activities help the client progress by easy stages from the task at which he is most likely to succeed—evaluation of another speaker's production—through the intermediate stages of evaluation of recorded speech, to the crucial but most difficult task of evaluating his own production during the speaking act.

Step 1. The clinician produces three sounds or syllables or words. They may all be correct or may include some errors, such as [iɚ], [iɚ], [iə]. Clients evaluate the productions by stating that all are correct or all are not correct. In the latter case, clients must be able to state which productions were not acceptable, number one, number two, or number three. In the above example, number three would be identified as the error. The clinician rewards correct evaluations. Here the client discriminates between correct and error productions in the speech of another speaker.

Step 2. The clinician records a group of three productions on tape, either correct or demonstrating errors. Clients evaluate the clinician's productions on playback, again as in Step 1, identifying any errors by number. The clinician rewards correct evaluations. Here the client engages in discrimination of another person's speech production, recorded instead of live.

Step 3. The clinician produces a single utterance, which the client tries to imitate. Both productions are recorded and played back. The client judges whether his production sounded the same as that of the model. Here the client is judging his own utterance and that of the model under the same airborne condition. At first, the clinician rewards the client's correct evaluation even though production may be defective. Later in the process, both correct evaluation and production are rewarded.

Step 4. The clinician produces a group of three utterances, such as [ber], [ber], [ber]. The client attempts to match them, likewise producing three consecutive utterances. The model and the imitation are tape-recorded and played back for evaluation by the client.

At first, the clinician rewards precision of evaluation—that is, the client must be able to tell whether all of his productions matched those of the model or, if not consistently correct, which were defective, number one, number two, or number three. The task is more demanding than evaluation of his own single production.

Later, both correct evaluation and production are rewarded. Here again, the client is monitoring his own voice along with that of the model as though both were voices of other speakers. However, he is in fact tuning in to his own production with precision.

Step 5. The client records three utterances on tape without a model. On playback, he evaluates his own productions, identifying errors by number.

At first, the clinician rewards only correct evaluation. Later, both correct evaluation and production are rewarded. In this task, the client is coming closer to evaluation of his production simultaneous with utterance, since in the latter instance, he will have no model but the internalized standard.

Step 6. The client records three utterances on tape without a model. He is required to listen carefully to his productions during the act of speaking. He must make a judgment about correctness or error *prior* to playback, identifying any errors by number. He then listens to the same productions on playback and evaluates them in the same precise fashion. Subsequently, he compares the two judgments. If he determines, upon listening to playback, that his judgment based on simultaneous auditory feedback was not accurate, he will realize that he was not sufficiently tuned in to his production during the act of speaking. This realization motivates a heightened level of self-monitoring on subsequent attempts, the cumulative effect of which tends to develop a highly refined auditory feedback mechanism which eventually serves to monitor production of the newly acquired [r] phoneme in running speech.

The implementing device for Step 6 is a score sheet (fig. 36), composed of two columns. The scoring procedure is based on

SELF-LISTENING SCORE SHEET

Place a V on a line if all target sounds in a response are judged correct.

Place an X on a line if all target sounds in a response are *not* judged correct.

Record each response on tape. Judge the same response before and after playback.

In Column I, place a V or X representing judgments made *during* each speech response *before* hearing playback of recorded production.

In Column II, place a V or X representing judgments made *after* hearing the same production on playback of recorded speech.

Compare the two sets of judgments, appearing side by side, next to the same numbers in the two columns. Repeat the activity until at least 80 percent or 8 pairs of judgments are the same in both columns.

	Trial 1, date _____		Trial 2, date _____		Trial 3, date _____	
	Col. I	Col. II	Col. I	Col. II	Col. I	Col. II
1.	_____	_____	_____	_____	_____	_____
2.	_____	_____	_____	_____	_____	_____
3.	_____	_____	_____	_____	_____	_____
4.	_____	_____	_____	_____	_____	_____
5.	_____	_____	_____	_____	_____	_____
6.	_____	_____	_____	_____	_____	_____
7.	_____	_____	_____	_____	_____	_____
8.	_____	_____	_____	_____	_____	_____
9.	_____	_____	_____	_____	_____	_____
10.	_____	_____	_____	_____	_____	_____

Fig. 36. Self-listening score sheet

the principle of error-signal detection. Clients make an appropriate mark indicating either that all productions in the group were correct or that all were not correct. Evaluations based upon judgments made during the speaking act are placed in Column I, and those made as a result of listening to playback of the recorded utterances are placed in Column II in spaces directly adjacent to the scoring spaces in Column I.

Therapy can employ an automatic playback tape recorder, such as the Echorder. With such a device, which provides playback at various preselected time intervals, judgment of production in playback can immediately succeed judgment of production during utterance. In this case, a client will say item 1, score it in Column I, hear it in playback, and score it in the adjacent line in Column II.

With a conventional recorder, the entire Column I can be marked first, and then folded under so that the markings are out of sight. Then playback of all items are rated in Column II. The paper is then unfolded, and the scores in the two columns are compared.

Should clients fail to produce the sounds correctly and/or identify their error productions on any particular level, move back to the previous step. If difficulty persists, repeatedly replay the recorded item(s), directing the client's attention to specific instances and/or features of the error production. In cases where the auditory feedback alone is not effective, attention may be directed to visual and/or tactile cues in conjunction with vivid verbal imagery—for example, "Look in the mirror. Is your 'gate' open or closed? Is your tongue 'upstairs' or 'downstairs'? Is your tongue like a 'pillow' or like a 'board'?"

These procedures and the following materials were designed for use in a research program which investigated their effectiveness in achieving carryover of the [r] allophones to spontaneous speech (Gerber 1966). Results demonstrated that the experimental group, trained with this program, achieved a significantly higher incidence of carryover than the control group, trained with more traditional methods. The principle studied was the comparative effects of intrapersonal versus interpersonal auditory feedback.

8

THE PROGRAM

T HE stimuli in this program progress from tasks involving production of the stressed syllabic (or vocalic) [ɝ] to production of other allophones. Since [ɝ] is a steady-state vowel, it provides, in prolonged form, sufficient time to achieve the conditions necessary for production and, at the same time, adequate opportunity to evaluate that production auditorily.

The materials are presented in eight levels of complexity, ranging from the more structured to the relatively spontaneous response. After successful production of one level of material at a slow rate, the client repeats the same material at a more rapid rate. A performance that is 80 percent successful at the speed of running speech is the criterion for progress to the next level. At a slow rate, the [r] is somewhat prolonged, so that the client has a chance to "taste" the sound and to tune in to the quality of production. On more rapid attempts, production should be natural, devoid of exaggerated prolongation. The therapeutic process herein involved is one that moves the client toward articulation within conditions as similar as possible to those of spontaneous speech. Concurrently, the ability to monitor increasingly rapid production is fostered.

LEVELS OF MATERIAL

Level 1

This level consists of simple syllables which progress from production achieved with a high probability of success to the next level of difficulty.

As stated above, the stressed vocalic [ɝ] is used as a pivot, from which other allophones are shaped. It is presented intervocalically (e.g., [eɝe]) in order to provide discernible movement to and from the [r] position. This intervocalic position is then modified in two directions. First, by deletion of the second vowel, it becomes the postvocalic [r] in the final position [eɝ]. Deletion of the first vowel yields [ɝ] in a prevocalic initial position [ɝe]. By a gradual increase of the speed of sequences of these syllables, the steady-state vowel is reduced to the consonantal [re].

Although all the allophones, with the exception of the prevocalic blend, are presented on Level 1, I do not recommend that all categories be worked on concurrently. Instead, I suggest that the stressed vocalic [ɝ] be stabilized in both the intervocalic context (e.g., [eɝe]) and in the CV syllable (e.g., [bɝ]). The [ɝ] is presented in the closed C[ɝ]C syllable as well. As the client progresses from the open C[ɝ] syllable to closure with the arresting consonant, I suggest that the [ɝ] be prolonged until the client is certain of its production. Only then, in response to a cue from the clinician, should the final consonant be added. Moving from these, I have found the probability of the greatest success in the postvocalic position (e.g., [eɝ]), combining the [ɝ] with the front vowels only, until production is well established. Premature combination with back vowels [ɔ] and [u] frequently results in distortion of [r] quality; such combinations should be reserved until a high degree of stabilization has been achieved.

Production of the prevocalic glide (e.g., [re]), the unstressed vocalic [ɚ], and the postvocalic preconsonantal offglides (e.g., [ɔɚd]) should be deferred until the first three allophones have been stabilized on Levels 1, 2, and 3. Only after this cumulative mastery of the easier allophones has been accomplished should an attack be made on the more difficult allophones at Level 1.

The above suggestion will not pertain to all cases. Some clients possess the consonantal glide but have not developed the vocalic allophones. The reverse is true for others. Still others may respond unpredictably to stimulation, thereby indicating completely different priorities. The recommendations concerning order of attack is based upon behavior manifested by most, but not all, cases I have encountered.

The syllables are presented orally, at first, by the clinician. The client responds in the manner described in the six steps of the self-monitoring training program above, striving simultaneously for consistency of production and precision of evaluation at increasing levels of speed.

Stressed Syllabic

bɝ bɝ bɝb

dɝ dɝ dɝd

fɝ fɝ fɝf

kɝ kɝ kɝk

pɝ pɝ pɝp

Postvocalic Final

eɝe eɝ eɝ

iɝi iɝ iɝ

aɪɝaɪ aɪɝ aɪɝ

ɔɝɔ ɔɝ ɔɝ

aɝa aɝ aɝ

Prevocalic Glide

eɝe ɝe ɝe

iɝi ɝi ɝi

aɪɝaɪ ɝaɪ ɝaɪ

oɝo ɝo ɝo

uɝu ɝu ɝu

Unstressed Syllabic

æbɚ æbɚ tæbɚ

æfɚ æfɚ kæfɚ

ækɚ ækɚ vækɚ

æpɚ æpɚ sæpɚ

ætɚ ætɚ kætɚ

Postvocalic Preconsonantal

ɔɚ ɔɚ ɔɚb

ɔɚ ɔɚ ɔɚd

ɔɚ ɔɚ ɔɚs

ɔɚ ɔɚ ɔɚk

ɔɚ ɔɚ ɔɚt

aɚ aɚ aɚd

aɚ aɚ aɚg

aɚ aɚ aɚk

aɚ aɚ aɚn

aɚ aɚ aɚt

Level 2

At this level, the client proceeds from production in nonsense words to production in meaningful words that are minimally contrastive—that is, only one phoneme has been added to, or changed in, the nonsense word to construct the English word. The client is required to produce the same correct [r] in the meaningful words as was produced in the nonsense with which it is paired—for example, sare, sare, care.

As in Level 1, practice progresses through the six steps of the self-monitoring training program. Proficiency at a slow rate of speed allows the client to repeat the material at faster rates until he is consistent in production and evaluation at the speed of running speech, with three units uttered on one breath.

Postvocalic Final

sare	sare	care
keer	keer	beer
pire	pire	tire
vore	vore	door
garr	garr	car

Stressed Syllabic

ferb	ferb	first
therk	therk	third
werp	werp	word
lert	lert	learn
berf	berf	bird

Initial Prevocalic [r]

rabe	rabe	rake
rees	rees	reed
rike	rike	ride
rofe	rofe	rode
rupe	rupe	rude

Blends

pree	pro	pray
cree	cro	cray
dree	dro	dray
free	fro	fray
gree	gro	gray

Unstressed Syllabic

lister	lister	sister
bunder	bunder	under
mather	mather	lather
saker	saker	baker
ketter	ketter	better

Postvocalic Preconsonantal

ord	ord	cord	ard	ard	hard
ork	ork	fork	ark	ark	park
orm	orm	warm	arn	arn	barn
ors	ors	horse	arp	arp	harp
ort	ort	port	art	art	cart

Level 3

Level 3 consists of production of three meaningful words. Initially, the goal is consistent production and accurate evaluation at a careful rate, through the six steps in the self-monitoring training program. Ultimately, the objective is the production of three words on one breath in approximately one second.

Although the stimuli may be presented orally by the clinician during early stages of practice, the words may eventually be read by clients who are capable of doing so.

Initial Prevocalic [r]			Blends		
rake	rake	rake	brown	brown	brown
rain	rain	rain	crown	crown	crown
rake	rain	rake	brown	crown	brown
reed	reed	reed	dry	dry	dry
reach	reach	reach	fry	fry	fry
reed	reach	reed	dry	fry	dry
ride	ride	ride	pray	pray	pray
ripe	ripe	ripe	gray	gray	gray
ride	ripe	ride	pray	gray	pray
rode	rode	rode	three	three	three
rose	rose	rose	free	free	free
rode	rose	rode	three	free	three
rude	rude	rude	try	try	try
roof	roof	roof	cry	cry	cry
rude	roof	rude	try	cry	try

Postvocalic Final			Syllabic Stressed [ɝ]		
care	care	care	first	first	first
bear	bear	bear	third	third	third
care	bear	care	first	third	first
deer	deer	deer	word	word	word
here	here	here	worm	worm	worm
deer	here	deer	word	worm	word
tire	tire	tire	turn	turn	turn
wire	wire	wire	burn	burn	burn
tire	wire	tire	turn	burn	turn
door	door	door	curl	curl	curl
more	more	more	furl	furl	furl
door	more	door	curl	furl	curl
car	car	car	bird	bird	bird
far	far	far	herd	herd	herd
car	far	car	bird	herd	bird

Postvocalic Preconsonantal

born	born	born	barn	barn	barn
corn	corn	corn	darn	darn	darn
born	corn	born	barn	darn	barn
cord	cord	cord	card	card	card
lord	lord	lord	yard	yard	yard
cord	lord	cord	card	yard	card
fork	fork	fork	park	park	park
pork	pork	pork	mark	mark	mark
fork	pork	fork	park	mark	park
port	port	port	part	part	part
fort	fort	fort	dart	dart	dart
port	fort	port	part	dart	part
horse	horse	horse	farm	farm	farm
morse	morse	morse	harm	harm	harm
horse	morse	horse	farm	harm	farm

Unstressed Syllabic

sister	sister	sister
mister	mister	mister
sister	mister	sister
other	other	other
mother	mother	mother
other	mother	other
better	better	better
letter	letter	letter
better	letter	better
madder	madder	madder
ladder	ladder	ladder
madder	ladder	madder
bolder	bolder	bolder
colder	colder	colder
bolder	colder	bolder

Level 4

The words listed in this level are presented by means of pictures drawn from the Warnock-Medlin Word-Making Kit. Here the letter stimulus is eliminated as a cue, and the words are more diverse in phonetic structure. Once again, the goal is utterance of three words on one breath at the speed of running speech. These words may consist of one word repeated or of three different words.

I strongly recommend that the six steps in the self-monitoring program be faithfully followed through Level 4. By this time, precision of self-evaluation has usually become highly developed. Thereafter, material is produced once instead of three times, and some of the early steps of self-monitoring are eliminated.

Prevocalic (I. and M.)		Postvocalic (F.)		Postvocalic Preconsonantal
arrow	ring	star	floor	corner
carrot	rolling pin	car	tire	arm
rooster	rake	bear	fire	corn
parrot	rain	deer	hair	horn
radio	rock	four	pear	barn
rabbit	merry-go-round	door	chair	heart
road	rowboat	jar		marbles
ruler	rug			sharpener
ribbon	giraffe			yarn
fairy	rattle			garden (yard)

Blends	Stressed Syllabic	Unstressed Syllabic	
brother	curtain	tiger	iron
cracker	girl	butter	hammer
umbrella	curls	letter	spider
crib	nurse	flower	corner
frog	turtle	water	lantern
truck	shirt	zipper	doctor
bridge	squirrel	scissors	mirror
drum	church	razor	woodpecker
broom	thermos	freezer	rooster
fruit	purse	shower	mother
train		teacher	father
bread		pitcher	mixer
trunk		collar	watermelon
brush			
crayon			

Level 5

Here functional units of speech are presented at a simple level. The prevocalic singles and blends and the unstressed syllabic [ɚ] are included in carrier sentences. The stressed syllabic [ɝ] and the postvocalic final and preconsonantal [r]'s are included in easy arithmetic activities. Communicative content is increased but controlled.

Once again, production should be consistent and accurately monitored at a careful rate before proceeding to the rate of natural running speech. Occasionally, clients are able to produce and monitor these units at a more rapid rate without the necessity of slow articulation. The clinician will of course determine at which level the client is able to maintain correct production and accurate self-evaluation. I strongly urge that the level of simultaneous auditory feedback be rigorously maintained, using a device such as the scoring sheet (or something similar), since, as communicative content gradually increases, the client's natural tendency is to divert attention from the articulation to the meaning of the utterance.

Prevocalic (Singles and Blends)
I like Ruth, but I don't like Ricky.
I like Robert, but I don't like Bruce.
I like Richard, but I don't like Brenda.
I like Robin, but I don't like Craig.
I like Rose, but I don't like Grace.
I like Ralph, but I don't like Mary.
I like Rita, but I don't like Karen.

Unstressed Syllabic
Add "er" to the last word in the following sentences:

He's late.	It's old.
He's big.	It's new.
He's small.	She's fat.
It's cold.	She's young.
It's hot.	She's slow.
It's soft.	She's wise.
It's white.	She's thin.

Number Activities

1. Count from 30 to 39. $[\,ɝ\,]$
2. Count from 40 to 49. $[\,ɔɝ\,t\,]$
3. Say the 3-times table. (prevocalic blend)
4. Say the 4-times table. $[\,ɔɝ\,]$
5. Say the following arithmetic examples aloud:

```
    4          4          7          0
  + 0        × 4        − 3      10 ⟌ 00
  ───        ───        ───
    4         16          4
```

```
    3         10         13          4
  + 4        × 3        − 4      10 ⟌ 40
  ───        ───        ───
    7         30          9
```

```
    9          9         11          4
  + 4        × 4        × 4       4 ⟌ 16
  ───        ───        ───
   13         36         44
```

```
   10         34         44         13
  + 4        − 4       − 40       4 ⟌ 52
  ───        ───        ───
   14         30          4
```

```
    4         10         34         13
  − 4        × 4        − 4       3 ⟌ 39
  ───        ───        ───
    0         40         30
```

Level 6

This level presents short, simple sentences for each of the allo-phones. (See Part I, above, for similar kinds of sentences for the young child.) By this time, if all procedures have been carefully followed, there should be no need for slow, careful production. The sentences should be spoken or read at the natural rate of running speech with normal patterns of rhythm and intonation. I believe that the all too common practice of allowing (or even, in some cases, encouraging) clients to utter sentences in stilted, laborious fashion actually interferes with the achievement of carryover.

At this point, as in Level 5, rigorous standards for self-evalua-tion should accompany the more complex production tasks, to insure effective feedback during subsequently more communica-tive speech. Tape recording should continue to be used through-out all levels.

Initial Prevocalic (Single)
1. The boy ran away.
2. I see a rose.
3. The rose is red.
4. Sue is playing the radio.
5. Can you read?
6. I will race you.
7. She has a pet rabbit.
8. Give me a ride.
9. Run up the hill.
10. Can you jump rope?

Prevocalic Blends
1. The tree is big.
2. I have a frog.
3. The crow flew away.
4. The grass is green.
5. Dick won the prize.
6. He is my friend.
7. You have brown eyes.
8. I like that dress.
9. The baby is in the crib.
10. We went on a train.

Intervocalic
1. Pat is very tall.
2. Carry the baby.
3. I don't like carrots.
4. Mary wants to play.
5. I'm sorry he is sick.
6. Hurry to school.
7. She sang a merry song.
8. Harry went home.
9. We picked berries.
10. Tell me a story.

Postvocalic, Final Position
1. He has a flat tire.
2. They have a blue car.
3. Jane has nice hair.
4. We saw a deer.
5. Do you see a bear?
6. Open the door.
7. Sit on the chair.
8. The star shines.
9. Here is the book.
10. I have four cats.

Postvocalic, Preconsonantal
1. That horse can jump.
2. Come to the park.
3. Mommy is tired.
4. Blow the horn.
5. He lives on a farm.
6. Play in the yard.
7. My fork fell down.
8. The pig ate the corn.
9. My arm is tired.
10. The barn is white.

Stressed Vocalic Syllabic
1. The bird flew away.
2. John is first in line.
3. The lady is a nurse.
4. Take a turn.
5. Can you say this word?
6. The girl went home.
7. I found a worm.
8. We heard a noise.
9. Let's dig in the dirt.
10. My turtle died.

Unstressed Vocalic Syllabic
1. We ate dinner.
2. Mother sang a song.
3. My father is big.
4. I need a ladder.
5. The water is cold.
6. Hammer the nail.
7. Cover the baby.
8. I picked a flower.
9. He has a better one.
10. I mailed the letter.

Level 7

All the allophones of [r] are included in each of the paragraphs used here. They are of course to be read with natural prosody. Avoid the stilted, artificial patterns characteristic of so much reading. No slow rate of production is employed at this level. Both articulation and monitoring are carried out at the speed of running speech. Tape recording is indispensable for the detection of errors in the complex context.

It is obvious that the reading level is above that of the young child. Many children at the second grade level can, however, with much repetition of a model, learn to read the passage, almost by rote. Those in third grade or higher should generally have no difficulty.

The Brown Family

The Brown family lives on a farm. It is a very large family. There are the mother and father. There are three sisters and four brothers. Their names are Ruth, Martha, Shirley, Robert, Richard, Gordon, and Arthur. Each of the children has his own horse. The girls have pet birds. The boys have pet turtles. They raise flowers and vegetables in their garden. They grow roses, carnations, and asters. They also raise carrots, radishes, and cucumbers. Mr. Brown raises corn and barley. They all work hard but are very happy.

The Green Family

The Green family lives in the heart of town. They are not a large family. There are the mother and father. There are the sister and brother. Their names are Margaret and Peter. They live in an apartment. There are four rooms on the fourteenth floor. They drive to school in a car pool. They play in a park across the street. They buy their clothes at the department store. Mr. Green works in a skyscraper. Mrs. Green has a washer, a dryer, and a dishwasher. Life here is very different from life on a farm.

Level 8

This level elicits responses most closely approximating spontaneous speech, in that no visual (letter) cues are offered and in that replies involve concentration of attention on content to a degree that shifts much of the focus away from articulation. It is expected that these responses will be uttered in completely spontaneous fashion and that the simultaneous auditory feedback mechanism will be functioning at an almost automatic level. Comparisons of clients' judgments during speech and during playback of the recorded production (on the score sheet) are crucial at this level, to insure the fact that self-monitoring can function to maintain the corrected sound under conditions similar to those of the terminal behavior.

Procedures

1. Tell the client that he will be asked questions that present choices. He is to answer each question in a complete sentence, incorporating one of the two alternatives in his response.
2. The clinician reads a question. The client records his response on tape and marks his judgment of the [r] production in Column I of the self-listening score sheet.
3. The response is played back, and the client marks his judgment of the recorded production in Column II of the self-listening score sheet.

The questions are read aloud to the client, who answers in complete sentences at normal speaking rate with natural intonation.

Prevocalic

1. Do rabbits like carrots or radishes?
2. Would you rather have roast beef or roast chicken?
3. Shall I wear a ribbon or a rose in my hair?
4. Did she have a ruby ring or a diamond ring?
5. Was the answer right or wrong?
6. Shall I give the ruler to Ruth or Richard?
7. Shall we play Red Rover or Run Sheep Run?
8. Is the radio in the dining room or the living room?
9. Is that a robin or a wren in the tree?
10. Shall we meet at the railroad station or at the river?

Blends

1. Is she wearing a green dress or a brown dress?
2. Do you want your fish fried or broiled?
3. Is the fruit fresh or frozen?
4. Would you say it's pretty good or pretty bad?
5. Did you practice the crawl stroke or the breast stroke?
6. Will you be driving or going by train?
7. Shall we trick or treat or just dress up?
8. Did you say Grandmother broke her thread or her bread?
9. Who was heartbroken, the prince or the princess?
10. Did Bruce sleep in a cradle or in a crib?

Postvocalic (F.)

1. Did you see a bear or deer?
2. Did you paint the door or the chair?
3. Is the car far or near?
4. Did you lose the jar here or there?
5. Did you cut your hair or your ear?
6. Did you buy a tire or some wire?
7. Do you or don't you care about the fair?
8. Shall I meet you at the drug store or the food store?
9. Are you sure or aren't you sure about the bus fare?
10. Are there four, or are there more than four?

Postvocalic Preconsonantal

1. Shall we go to the park or the farm?
2. Does he own fourteen horses or forty horses?
3. Is that Mark's cart or Morton's cart?
4. Did you park the car at the market or on the parking lot?
5. Is Marcia on the porch or in the garden?
6. Did you come before the storm or after the storm?
7. Does a deer have short horns or long horns?
8. Is your party March fourth or March twenty-fourth?
9. Shall we meet at the corner or at Gordon's house?
10. Do you want an apple tart or a lemon tart?

Stressed Syllabic

1. Is that a bird or a squirrel?
2. Did the big girl or the little girl get dirty?
3. Is the worm in the earth or on the earth?
4. Did you misspell the first word or the third word?
5. Is the purse hers or yours?
6. Whose sunburn was worse, Burt's or Gert's?
7. Is it Myrtle's turn or Kurt's turn?
8. Were there thirty or thirty-five girls?
9. Is that dirt or a burn on your arm?
10. Is the turtle named Gertie or Bertie?

Unstressed Syllabic

1. Would you rather go over or under the bridge?
2. Who came with you, your father or your mother?
3. Did you go with your sisters or your brothers?
4. Are they older or younger than you?
5. Do you add some flour or some butter to the batter?
6. Is your birthday in summer or in winter?
7. Did you buy a hammer or a ladder?
8. Shall I move it higher or lower?
9. Would you rather wear a sweater or a blazer?
10. Would you rather wear slippers or sneakers?

REFERENCES

REFERENCES

Arnold, G. 1956. A study of the value of amplified headphone listening and immediate playback in the correction of functional articulatory defects. *Speech Monographs*, 23, 137. Abstract of thesis, University of Houston. University Microfilms 14236.

Aufricht, H. 1960. A comparison of the listening skills of 65 children with articulatory defects and a matched group of children with normal speech. *Speech Monographs*, 27, 153. Abstract of thesis, Northwestern University.

Aungst, L., and Frick, J. V. 1964. Auditory discrimination ability and consistency of articulation of [r]. *Journal of Speech and Hearing Disorders* 29: 76-85.

Carrell, J. A. 1968. *Disorders of articulation*. Englewood Cliffs, N.J.: Prentice-Hall.

Curtis, J. F., and Hardy, J. C. 1959. A phonetic study of misarticulation of [r]. *Journal of Speech and Hearing Research* 2: 244-57.

Gerber, A. J. 1966. The achievement of [r] carryover through intensification of simultaneous auditory feedback. *Pennsylvania Speech and Hearing Association Newsletter* VII.

Judson, L. S., and Weaver, A. T. 1942. *Voice science.* New York: Appleton-Century-Crofts.

McDonald, E. T. 1964. Articulation testing and treatment: A sensory-motor approach. Pittsburgh: Stanwix House.

Milisen, R., and assoc. 1954. The disorder of articulation: A systematic and clinical approach. *Journal of Speech and Hearing Disorders,* monograph supplement 4.

Mowrer, D. E. 1970. An analysis of motivational techniques used in speech therapy. *ASHA* 12: 491-93.

Mowrer, D. E.; Baker, R. J.; and Owen, C. 1968. Verbal content analysis of speech therapy sessions. Paper presented at the annual convention of the American Speech and Hearing Association, Denver.

Shames, G. H. 1957. Use of the nonsense syllable in articulation therapy. *Journal of Speech and Hearing Disorders* 22: 261-63.

Sommers, R. K. 1969. Problems in therapy. In *Clinical speech in the schools,* ed. R. J. Van Hattum. Springfield, Ill.: Charles C. Thomas.

Van Riper, C. 1963. *Speech correction: Principles and methods.* 4th ed. Englewood Cliffs, N.J.: Prentice-Hall.

Van Riper, C., and Irwin, J. V. 1958. *Voice and articulation.* Englewood Cliffs, N.J.: Prentice-Hall.

Winitz, H. 1969. *Articulatory acquisition and behavior.* New York: Appleton-Century-Crofts.

Wright, V.; Shelton, R. L.; and Arndt, W. B. 1969. A task for evaluation of articulation change: III. Imitative task scores compared with scores for more spontaneous tasks. *Journal of Speech and Hearing Research* 12: 875-83.